Walk the Talk
First Responder Peer Support

A Boots-on-the-Ground Peer and Trauma Support Systems Guide

By
Staff Sergeant (Ret'd) Brad McKay
and
Staff Sergeant (Ret'd) Sylvio (Syd) A. Gravel, M.O.M.

Syd A. Gravel/Budd Publishing
Ottawa, Ontario

Copyright by Sylvio (Syd) A. Gravel, M.O.M., and Brad McKay, 2016

Published by: Syd A. Gravel/Budd Publishing

URL: www.56secondsbook.com

Library and Archives Canada Cataloguing in Publication

McKay, Brad, 1959-, author

   "Walk the talk" first responder peer support / Brad McKay, Sylvio Gravel.

Issued in print and electronic formats.
ISBN 978-0-9881316-6-8 (paperback). —ISBN 978-0-9881316-7-5 (pdf)

     1. First responders—Job stress. 2. First responders—Psychology. 3. Employee health promotion. 4. Stress management. I. Gravel, Sylvio A., 1952-, author II. Title.

RC963.48.M35 2016	158.7'2	C2016-901600-5
		C2016-901601-3

Electronic monograph in PDF format.
Issued in print format.
Cover photo: Heidi Garrison
Sketches: Erin McKay and Drew Dunning
Cover and Book Design: Budd Publishing
Editor: Eleanor Sawyer

All rights reserved. Without limiting the rights under the copyright reserved above, no part of this publication may be reproduced, stored in or introduced into a database and retrieval system or transmitted in any form or by any means (electronic, mechanical, photocopying, recording or otherwise) without the prior written permission of both owners of copyright and the above-noted publisher.

PRINTED IN CANADA

Contents

Foreword vii
Preface ix
Acknowledgments xi

1—Protecting Society's Protectors through Peer Support 1
    Dealing with the Stigma of Mental Disorders 3
    How an Organization Can Care for Its Employees' Mental Health Needs 8

2—Assessing an Organization's Awareness about Workplace Wellness 13

3—Getting Management Onside 19
    Setting Up the Action Committee 19
    Addressing the Ten Key Issues 20

4—Organizational Pre-Hiring Preparedness 35
    At the Pre-Hiring Stage 36
    On Being Hired 37

5—Organizational Support for Families 41
    Failing the Family 41
    What the Organization Can Do 45
    The Importance of a Family Relationship 46

6—Middle Management Leadership 51
    Building Trust 51
    Training Middle Managers 52
    Effective Tools for Middle Management 54
    Suicide Awareness 55

Contents

7—Developing a Critical Incident Stress Management (CISM) Team 59
    The CISM Model 59
    Developing a CISM Team 61
    The Multidisciplinary CISM Team 62
    Deployment of the CISM Team 64
    Controversy and an Optional Approach 65

8—Developing Peer Support Teams 67
    Peer Support from Syd Gravel's Experience 67
    The Legitimacy of Informal Peer Support 69
    Psychological Testing 74
    Peer Support from Brad McKay's Experience 75
    A Caution about Social Media 78
    Formal Peer Support Teams 79
    CISM versus Peer Support 79
    Peer Support Alone 81

9—Staffing CISM and Peer Support Teams 83
    Getting Started 83
    Staffing the Team 87
    Additional Peer Support Members 95

10—Organizational Training for CISM and Peer Support Teams 99
    Organizational Training Resources 100

11—How a CISM and Peer Support System Can Work 111
    Selecting Strategies and Tools 111
    Psychological Services 120

12—Walking the Talk 125

13—Brad's Story 127
    The Trauma Event 127
    The Aftermath 130
    Developing a Peer Support Network 132
    Where I Am Today 136

14—Syd's Story 139
The Lead-Up 139
The Trauma Event 142
The Aftermath 145
The Downward Spiral 147
Personal Reaction and Spousal Support 149
The Moral Injury 151
Peer Support 154
Where I Am Today 155

Notes 159
About the Authors 167
What Others Are Saying 171

Foreword

As a psychotherapist with over thirty years of experience, peer support has played an integral role in my trauma practice. Whether through individual or group support, peer supporters have helped to save families, careers and the lives of their coworkers.

Walk the Talk is an invitation for the reader to discover the rationale for, and the development and implementation of, an effective peer support program. Such a program can be instrumental in mitigating the negative consequences of traumatic events within an organization, particularly first responder services or agencies.

As a result of their own boots-on-the-ground experience of an operational stress injury, retired Staff Sergeants Brad McKay and Syd Gravel have each walked the road of recovery. Through their own learning and post-traumatic growth, their personal lives and careers were enhanced as they used their own experiences, insights and training to introduce informal and formal peer support programs to their own police services in order to assist their injured colleagues.

We know that humans are social beings who need to connect and share with others. We are also aware that life situations that create threats, pain and distress can lead to suffering—often suffering in silence. Isolation, loneliness and a lack of support increase the negative consequences of traumatic events in our lives and directly impact our brain's health. In addition, there is a relationship between exposure to trauma, post-traumatic stress disorder (PTSD) and chronic medical conditions. All of these can create an emotional, physical and financial cost to an organization.

The practices outlined in this book are evidence-based, with the training of peers using the seventeen evidenced-based modules that follow the guidelines set by the Mental Health Commission of Canada, and which are endorsed and supported by the Mood Disorders Society of Canada.

The authors have outlined step-by-step procedures to help an organization identify its needs and select the leaders who will have credibility in a peer support program. Both authors are passionate and knowledgeable speakers, and advocates of the importance of peer support in mental health recovery.

With the tools in this book as a template, an organization now has the means to implement a peer support program that clearly states to its employees that the organization wants to prevent complications after traumatic events and strengthen resilience. The organization will be ready to "walk the talk" for mental health.

Barbara Anschuetz, EdD, RP, CTSS
Registered Psychotherapist

Preface

As the final touches were being put on this book, there were nine suicides among frontline responders in Canada in the first five weeks of 2016. Seven of them were in Ontario.[1] For those who have been a first responder, one suicide is too many.

Suicide does not need to happen. There are risk factors that can be identified, and peers who can be trained to assist in identifying these factors before something bad happens within an organization, especially first responder services such as police, fire, paramedic and health care emergency departments.

Research shows that eighty percent of suicides have a degree of pre-communication before the act is completed.[2] Therefore, organizations have a responsibility to protect their employees from committing harmful or life-threatening acts against themselves, or possibly others, as a consequence of experiencing ongoing trauma resulting from their jobs. Organizations need the tools to provide assistance and support and not just tools to react to members' needs. Additional tools and resources are available to create a proactive system of early intervention that provides support and resources to employees before they become lost in a hole of despair.

Both authors have experienced trauma on the job and understand what can lead to thoughts of suicide and how tempting it can be as a solution for someone who is suffering from trauma and believes there is no one to turn to for help.

Preface

Early intervention is the key to a shorter path to wellness, particularly mental wellness. The good news is that an organization can have a boots-on-the-ground peer support system that works. This book describes how to provide such a system through processes that are relatively easy to set up and relatively inexpensive to implement. Step by step, and chapter by chapter, the organization will learn about the information needed and the tools and resources available to build a competent and trusted peer support system.

The two authors have a combined total of fifty-five years of peer support experience. They understand the challenges and have overcome the hurdles in setting up peer support systems for their organizations and for other similar services.

They share their knowledge in this book, based on having walked the talk, in order to help others get started in implementing a peer support system.

Acknowledgments

The authors wish to acknowledge the contributions of the following organizations for the resources, workshops, documents and other sources that have been cited and/or directly quoted in this book, especially in chapter 10. The intent is to provide the reader with information that can be accessed quickly.

Nevertheless, documentation, workshops, surveys and other information cited here is the exclusive property of these organizations and all rights are reserved to them:

Association of Traumatic Stress Specialists (ATSS), Greenville, South Carolina

Badge of Life Canada

Canadian Centre for Occupational Health and Safety, Hamilton, Ontario

Canadian Critical Incident Stress Foundation
Hamilton, Ontario

Canadian Standards Association
Ottawa, Ontario

The International Critical Incident Stress Foundation, Inc., Ellicott City, Maryland

LivingWorks Education, Calgary, Alberta

Acknowledgments

Mental Health Commission of Canada
Ottawa, Ontario

Mood Disorders Society of Canada
Guelph, Ontario

National Organization for Victim Assistance
(NOVA), Alexandria, Virginia

Simon Fraser University, Faculty of Health
Sciences, Vancouver, British Columbia

The Tema Conter Memorial Trust
King City, Ontario

The Trauma Centre, Sharon, Ontario

York Regional Police, Aurora, Ontario

The York Region Critical Incident Stress Management
Team, East Gwillimbury, Ontario

1

Protecting Society's Protectors through Peer Support

This book addresses the needs of first responder organizations in order to support their staff and employees, or members, who are expected to run into chaotic or dangerous situations. While everyone else is running toward shelter and safety, first responders, that is, police officers, firemen, paramedics, and emergency department nurses and physicians are expected to meet danger head on or deal with its aftermath or consequences.

These organizations' members, or staff, are considered the protectors and frontline responders during times of crisis. The community depends on them and sleeps well at night knowing they are out there. They are expected to be trained mentally, physically and emotionally to dive into difficult, challenging and dangerous situations in order to preserve the peace, to ensure the health and safety of others and to save lives in a community.

They are considered to be strong, resilient, highly skilled and very successful at doing what they do. Generally, these individuals would be described as results-driven, boots-on-the-ground, step-up-to-the-plate types, who get the job done no matter how difficult it may be and, often, despite the various personalities involved and events that occur.

Every so often, however, one of these real-life heroes will encounter an event, or a series of events, so powerful and fearful, so horrific and out of their control, that their own ability to cope will be compromised. Whichever way this situation comes at them, it's often more than they can handle and they fall. The scary part is that it's a hidden injury; it's not immediately evident to those interacting with these people, or even to the individuals themselves, that they have been impacted in an adverse way.

Society sometimes forgets that, although first responders are well-trained and willingly sacrifice themselves for the good of the community, they are only human. Society needs to be reminded that they are also husbands and wives, mothers and fathers, sons and daughters, and brothers and sisters. They do homework with their children, take out the garbage weekly, argue over dishes and have family holidays. They are like everyone else except they have been tasked with a huge responsibility and burden in their workplace. Yes, they are up for it and have agreed to face the unsavory duties asked of them because it's their job. They joined the organization knowing full well what was expected of them. But were they truly informed and prepared to face trauma after trauma, day in and day out?

In the course of an average individual's lifetime, a person may be confronted with one or two, possibly three, traumatic events at most. But in the first responder work environment, an individual can face between 600 to 850 traumatic events over the course of a career. How can a first responder know, or even understand, the short- and long-term impact of these traumatic events?

To do so, they need to be informed and given the tools to prepare for such events. The ability, knowledge and skills needed to understand and survive trauma are not achieved or learned simply through osmosis; considerable effort is required both on the part of first responders themselves and their organizations.

First responders are problem-solvers and are often viewed by society as an elite group—always strong, well prepared, never failing or faltering in their jobs. For the most part, they are able to maintain this image. However, as repeated exposure to trauma begins to take its toll and first responders show symptoms of a mental health injury, disorder or illness, this creates a significant barrier for them. They hesitate to take the first steps toward admitting they need help and are often unable to reach out for it, fearing both the stigma of appearing weak and the attitude surrounding mental health issues. First responder services need to understand what the impact is on their workforce of both the organization's and society's views on mental illness and the stigma it has created.

Dealing with the Stigma of Mental Disorders

The stigma of mental disorders is the most significant barrier to first responders getting the help and support they need.

In October 2012, the Ontario ombudsman released his report titled *In the Line of Duty*, which described how operational stress injuries were being handled for provincial police officers. In fact, the first recommendation in the report addresses the need for further measures to be taken by the police service to reduce the stigma of mental illness.[1] The report also included information about the attitudes within police services regarding mental health issues.

"Dr. John Violanti, [a renowned American expert in police suicide,] observed in July 2012 that the nature of the policing environment often goes against the goal of improving health."[2] He went on to state:

> The police culture doesn't look favorably on people who have problems.... Not only are you supposed to be superhuman if you're an officer, but you fear asking for help...... if you have heart disease, you may not be allowed to go back on the street.... That's a real threat. If you go for mental health counselling, you may not be considered for promotions and you may be shamed by your peers and superiors. In some cases, your gun can be taken away, so there's a real fear of going for help.[3]

In some police organizations, members on a stress-related leave may be ordered to turn in their badge and warrant card, which only increases the trauma for the officer.

The negative attitude toward those diagnosed with a mental illness or injury exists at all levels of organizations, services and agencies. This stigma against members or employees forces them to go underground where they battle their demons in isolation, confusion, fear and alone. If they do surface eventually to seek help, the road to recovery will be significantly longer than asking for help early on.

It takes courage to ask for help. For some, taking this first step is the most frightening thing they will ever do. For some who did seek help, they are not received well because those they trust and shared with are biased by the stigma. A negative experience like this may send the organization's members underground for long periods of time, possibly even years before they eventually attempt to seek help or are driven to do so by others.

The existing stigma also becomes a barrier for promotion or progression within their organization. Fear of being seen as weak or experiencing their own feelings of being unworthy forces the traumatized member or staff to hide their symptoms in order to avoid facing the stigma.

Sucking it up or toughing it out are terms used that encourage members to bottle up their mental health struggles. But there is a cost to untreated mental disorders and not just to the organization. There is a human cost as well both to employees and to their families, who often suffer the consequences when loved ones withdraw from them and isolate themselves.

In a Mental Health Commission of Canada survey, forty-six percent of respondents believed that mental illness was just an excuse for bad behaviour.[4] Canadian employers and employees were surveyed and respondents believed that a person experiencing depression would be less productive (65%) and would likely have to take extended sick leave (49%). They also believed that having a depressed coworker would affect the mood of all employees (42%), cost the company money (33%) and would make other employees uncomfortable (30%).

The stigma associated with a mental health disorder is not just confined to first responder organizations and services; bias and stigma are common all too often in every workplace. It is important that every organization have an anti-stigma campaign or strategy to address the need for all employees to know how to take care of their mental health and to know that doing so is a sign of strength not weakness. The importance of this type of initiative cannot be overemphasized.

As an example, the Mood Disorders Society of Canada has launched an anti-stigma campaign that encourages all organizations to deal with issues surrounding mental illness and the stigma in the workplace. It is called the Elephant in the Room; the organization provides posters for display in the workplace with the focus on raising awareness.

> When you **display** your blue elephant, you show that you care about the wellness of others and demonstrate that this is a safe place to talk about mental illness, without the fear of being viewed differently.
>
> When you see our little blue elephant, you know it's a safe place to speak about any mental health issues you or your family may be having. You will be treated with respect and dignity and you will find the support and understanding from a friend who cares.[5]

Reducing stigma in the workplace is everyone's responsibility. The organization can encourage mental health wellness and provide training opportunities for its staff to raise the level of

Photo 1.1 The Elephant in the Room

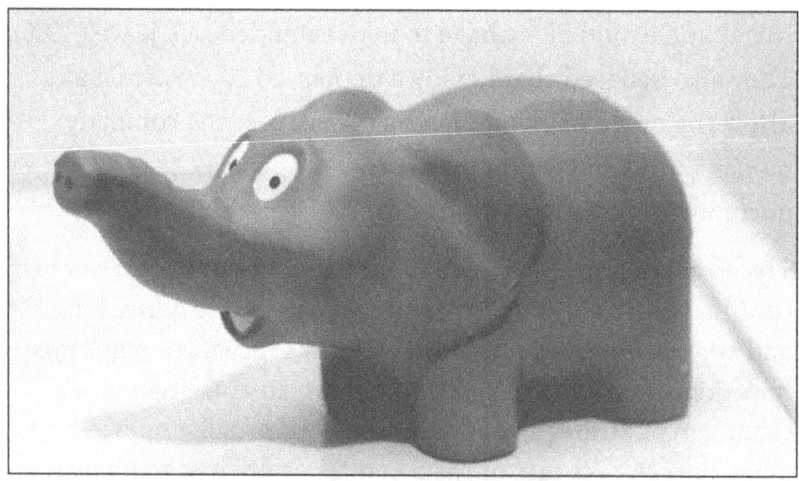

Source: http://www.mooddisorderscanada.ca/page/elephant-in-the-room-campaign

awareness in the workplace; these actions can be driven by the human resources and health and wellness departments. Communication from the CEO, or chief, can regularly include mental health wellness messages. The organization can also set aside a period of time each year as a mental health awareness opportunity to educate the workforce. The more awareness there is about mental health, the more likely people will lose the stigma against those with disorders.

Since 1951, the Canadian Mental Health Association has held Mental Health Week during the first week of May. The week is "a celebration of mentally healthy lifestyles and positive attitudes as well as a source of information and support."[6] An organization can adopt this week and use it as an awareness tool and training opportunity. It can bring in a respected guest speaker with a lived and survived mental health challenge to empower and inspire those employees, or members, who may need to reach out to someone.

In March 2016, the York Regional Police hosted an event and partnered with United by Trauma, the Barrie Police Service, the Ontario Provincial Police and the York and Barrie Police Associations to bring in a motivational speaker. Former NHL goaltender Clint Malarchuk discussed his struggle with addiction and PTSD. Events such as these effect change and reduce stigma across the organization. It is important to understand the impact of mental illness on the member and their family.

Many organizations offer a mental health awareness course. By showing employees that there are tools and resources available to deal with the issue of stigma, this will instill a sense of hope that recovery is possible. A trusted peer support team, with representatives from various ranks and/or levels of management within the organization can be tasked with delivering the message about mental health and anti-stigma campaigns.

Peers can also confront stigma head on through private and productive discussions with the old guard in the organization who still believe that everyone should just "suck it up" when struck by a traumatic impactful event or mental health challenge. A very frank, one-on-one, private discussion can help to turn these negative thoughts around. It will not be possible to change everyone's views or beliefs. But anyone exhibiting stigma behaviour should be confronted.

With everyone in the organization working together without stigma, the result will be a mentally healthier organization.

How an Organization Can Care for Its Employees' Mental Health Needs

When first responders do reach out, they need assurances that there are resources available and policies and procedures in place in their workplace for them to get the help and support they need in a timely fashion.

Old-school thoughts and approaches for dealing with mental health issues still prevail in many organizations today. But leading-edge organizations are taking a different view and fostering an environment of support in their workplace. They are now encouraging their staff, or members, to take care of their mental health. Reaching out for help is now seen as a sign of strength, not weakness.

It is not a simple undertaking for an organization to provide assistance and support for employees' or members' mental health needs. It isn't simply a matter of putting some procedures and policies, or resources, in place or providing training on a one-time basis. It is not that easy. Putting together some information sessions, providing employee assistance programs (EAPs) and a crisis intervention team to handle critical incidents are not enough when it comes to the mental health and safety of an organization's employees.

What good mental health management consists of is quietly, yet firmly, supporting and endorsing employees, or members, to take the lead in participating in whatever treatment and processes they know are best for them. They also need to know that they can seek treatment, support and therapy without any negative consequences to their employment status in the organization. It can be frightening to them if they think their injury or illness will jeopardize their current career or their future growth within the organization.

Ever since humankind has discovered the difference between sympathy and empathy, there has been informal peer support. There is always someone within the organization who has been in the same circumstances, especially a peer who has experienced something similar to what they are suffering. When members or employees fall, either through injury or illness, there is no one they will trust more than one of their own. Whether it is a trauma exposure while at work, or their child suddenly dying of cancer, there is significant value in the peer support provided by one of their own trusted members or colleagues, who has been there in difficult times, and whom they know will keep their vulnerability confidential.

Most significantly, the chief executive officer (CEO), president, general manager (GM) or chief has the ability to make decisions that could affect their employees' future in the organization. Simply put, an organization's members will take care of each other. But the response and support of both the CEO and senior management to the effects of trauma will strengthen this valuable resource of peer support within the workplace.

The organization may already have many levels of support in place. The CEO, chief or GM may be a compassionate leader who supports the members and employees. The human resources department may already have taken the lead in ensuring there are tools available. There may be an employee assistance program (EAP) offered, or a mental health professional to consult. The workplace may have excellent middle managers and supervisors who seek ways to improve the physical and mental well-being of their people and who watch for signs that an employee is having some mental health issues or showing signs of trauma.

Yet, despite all that has been done, the organization may still be struggling with mental health challenges, members booking off sick and incidents occurring in the workplace that indicate a lack of trust in management. There may also be conflicts or behavioural problems that challenge managers and supervisors, and take time away from their other duties. Worse yet, the organization may be trying to rebuild trust and confidence in the workplace environment after the suicide of one of its members or employees—the worst consequence of untreated trauma.

One important way in which an organization can protect its workforce and provide needed assistance, when its employees are experiencing the effects of a serious and potentially harmful trauma, is to provide a peer support system. Both informal and formal support systems can become primary tools within the organization.

The following chapters will describe the necessary steps that the organization can take to implement a peer support system.

2

Assessing an Organization's Awareness about Workplace Wellness

For an organization to move forward to provide a mentally healthy and safe work environment for their staff or members, the main question will be, Where does the organization start first?

There are tools available to determine the institutional level of awareness about workplace wellness. Most organizations should expect to find a wide range of awareness levels among individuals throughout the organization. It will no doubt be particularly revealing to discover how much variance there is in awareness, not only between but among the various levels of the workforce. The greater the variance the more complex the process will be to address the gaps in these awareness levels.

For the most part, the majority of first responder organizations have a level of awareness of workplace wellness that is at the unconscious incompetence stage. (*See* illustration 2.1 titled Conscious Competence Learning Matrix.) Through research and other resources, the organization can learn much more about educating its workforce to become more mentally healthy and aware of risk factors that act as barriers to moving forward. As more and more members of the organization increase their awareness, the organization will slowly move from the lower left quadrant of unconscious incompetence to conscious incompetence.

Illustration 2.1: Conscious Competence Learning Matrix

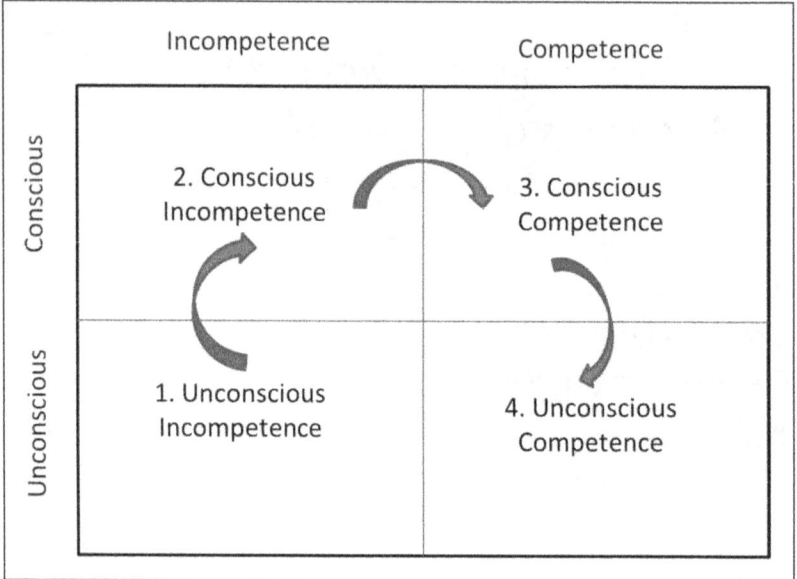

Source: The four stages of competence are taken from: http://en.wikipedia.org/wiki/Four stages of competence.

The organization needs to learn about the wealth of information now available to Canadian organizations, particularly since 2014. There has been considerable research and there are tools, workshops and other resources to assist organizations in creating mentally healthy and safe work environments.

A major first step for any organization is to become familiar with *Guarding Minds @ Work (GM@W)*.

> [This] is a unique and free, comprehensive set of resources designed to protect and promote psychological health and

safety in the workplace. GM@W resources allow employers to effectively assess and address the 13 psychosocial factors known to have a powerful impact on organizational health, the health of individual employees, and the financial bottom line. GM@W was developed by researchers from the Centre for Applied Research in Mental Health and Addiction (CARMHA) within the Faculty of Health Sciences at Simon Fraser University on the basis of extensive research, including data analysis of a national sample and reviews of national and international best practices, as well as existing and emerging Canadian case law and legislation.

GM@W is a response to current and emerging legal requirements in Canada for the protection of employee mental health and the promotion of civility and respect at work. Legal standards increasingly require employers to develop comprehensive strategies for ensuring a psychologically safe workplace. Prudent employers need to develop policies and programs that meet these new legal standards.

GM@W is available to all employers - large or small, in the public or private sector - at no cost. Workplaces may differ in the language describing various roles and positions. GM@W uses the terms "employee", "staff", "supervisor", "management" and "employer". [It is important to use the terms appropriate for your organization when reviewing the GM@W Assessment, Action and Evaluation Resources.][1]

Guarding Minds @ Work provides tools that will help the organization to make the argument to management about why it needs to create a psychologically healthy environment using business, legal, health, moral and/or ethical arguments to defend the need. This then becomes the business case to help move the organization forward to the next steps.

This program also offers tools to review and assess what may already exist such as policies and procedures, and occupational health and safety guidelines. It enables the organization to determine if there are any gaps between what is currently in place and what may be needed.

These tools also identify the thirteen psychosocial risk factors that need to be addressed in order to create a psychologically safe and healthy workplace. GM@W offers resources and survey tools to determine how the workforce views risk factors within the organization and how these may be addressed from their perspective. These tools enable the employer to see the difference between what exists and what should exist; what managers think exists and what employees see as existing. With this information in hand and available to everyone, it may now be possible for the organization to move forward.

After determining the employees' and management's perspectives, and identifying where the gaps are, the next step is how to address the psychosocial factors identified by GM@W.

The thirteen psychosocial risk factors "are elements that impact employees' psychological responses to work and work conditions, potentially causing psychological health problems."[2] These risk factors are:

> "PF1: Psychological Support
> PF2: Organizational Culture
> PF3: Clear Leadership & Expectations
> PF4: Civility & Respect
> PF5: Psychological Competencies & Requirements
> PF6: Growth & Development

PF7: Recognition & Reward

PF8: Involvement & Influence

PF9: Workload Management

PF10: Engagement

PF11: Balance

PF12: Psychological Protection [and]

PF 13: Protection of Physical Safety"[3]

Once all this information is made available to the organization, it can then shift to one that is ready to create change; the organization now knows how it is positioned in terms of its awareness of its psychological health and safety, or lack thereof, and what it must do to close the identified gaps and implement change. At this stage, the organization shifts to the conscious incompetence quadrant, which is the second stage of the learning matrix and where the organization and its staff are now positioned in terms of their level of awareness. Actions can now be taken to create the change needed to move forward to become psychologically healthy and safe. The goal should be to move to conscious competence.

In order to create the changes that must occur, it will need to look at another resource that is available to all organizations in Canada. This resource is the *National Standard of Canada for Psychological Health and Safety in the Workplace,* commonly known as the *Standard*. It was developed in 2013 by the Canadian Standards Association (CSA) and has been "championed by" the Mental Health Commission of Canada (MHCC). It is the first such standard of its kind in the world and focuses on employees' psychological health and safety exclusively.[4]

Along with the *Standard*, the CSA, in partnership with the MHCC, has also produced a guide on how to implement the standard in the workplace. This guide, *Assembling the Pieces: An Implementation Guide to the National Standard for Psychological Health and Safety in the Workplace*, was published in 2014.[5] This guide was developed in order to assist an organization wishing to implement the *Standard*.

Another key resource available to first responder organizations was published by the Mood Disorders Society of Canada in 2014. It is titled *Workplace Mental Health: How Employers Can Create Mentally Healthy Workplaces and Support Employees in Their Recovery from Mental Illness*.[6] This handbook provides a resource to create a mentally healthy workplace and also advises how it can support its workforce.

The task of creating change within an organization to meet the Canadian standards for psychological health and safety in the workplace can be daunting if attempted without using the documents identified in this chapter. It is not simply a matter of establishing new standards. All of these documents and tools provide guidelines and suggested actions to achieve the goal of ensuring a psychologically healthy and safe work environment.

Someone or some group in the organization now has to devote time and energy to creating the change needed to achieve the goal. The organization may want to strike a working committee to help manage the changes that have to occur with the ultimate goal being to create peer support teams in the organization.

3

Getting Management Onside

One of the more effective ways to implement change—and key to the entire process—is to get management at all levels of the organization onside.

Setting Up the Action Committee

A first step in bringing change and implementing trauma support systems is to set up the Trauma Support Systems Action Committee which should have the support of management. The title of the committee clearly conveys to everyone in the organization what its purpose is. Once the committee has been created, it is important to get a sense of what it will do to endorse and support the key components of trauma management, including peer-driven peer support programs.

The purpose of this committee is to address the following ten key issues for the organization. These are:

1. Selecting the lead person.
2. Selecting someone to champion the process.
3. Implementing the formal project management process.
4. Assessing the organizational need for trauma support systems.
5. Establishing the business case.

6. Researching best practices.
7. Determining the language to be used.
8. Creating a communications strategy.
9. Developing and supporting accessibility to resources.
10. Establishing a proactive approach through trauma support systems.

Addressing the Ten Key Issues

The Trauma Support Systems Action Committee is now responsible for addressing each of the following ten key issues.

KEY #1—SELECTING THE LEAD PERSON

The lead is that person within the organization who will work with management and the committee, as well as with all members in the workforce, to ensure that the committee's goals are attained. Most importantly, because of the nature of the change being implemented, the lead must be someone with a lived experience of trauma who is healthy and in an obvious positive stage of growth.

This person also has to have considerable personal power within the organization. The successful management of the Action Committee has very little to do with a person's positional power. It is much more to do with personal power, which by definition is the individual's personal stamina and ability to accomplish tasks in a passionately charged environment.

The most desirable person to lead a project, where change is required and emotions may be involved, is someone who has demonstrated strength, is highly respected, trusted and has a good understanding of the need for positional power to a varying degree. When there is a need for positional power the lead can call on the support of the champion. An example of this is when resources are required for the committee's work and these resources have to come from another section that is managed by someone in a senior executive position much higher than the position held by the lead. Personal power may not be enough to get that executive to agree to supply the resources needed; this is when the CEO, or the chief, can step in and ensure that the executive cooperates with the lead.

KEY # 2—SELECTING SOMEONE TO CHAMPION THE PROCESS

When a project involves complete organizational change, the champion has to be the most powerful person in the organization. If the chief executive officer (CEO), or the chief, doesn't buy into the process for trauma support systems and make it one of their priorities, then the project will go nowhere. No matter how big or small an organization the CEO has to champion the project and support the lead.

When delegating the champion role to anyone else but the CEO, other senior members of the management or executive team will likely view the project as belonging to someone else. They will probably dismiss it as nothing they have to pay attention to. It therefore becomes difficult to create the change that is required throughout the organization. If most members of the senior management team don't personally buy into the need for the trauma support systems project, at least, they may not do anything to hijack it, if the champion is the CEO.

The relationship between the project champion and the lead has to be one of mutual support. The champion may have to step in to open doors and remove obstructions. At other times, the lead will need to reassure the champion that the project is still moving in the right direction.

Successful projects may also attract attention from other organizations. Project leads are often asked to share their secrets in creating their trauma support systems. The most frequently asked questions are almost always the same: 1) How did you get the support and resources you needed? 2) How did you get the CEO on board? 3) How did you get the workforce (or the union/association) on board? 4) How did you deal with backlash in creating change? The response to all these questions is that the CEO was the project champion and onside throughout the implementation process.

KEY #3—IMPLEMENTING THE FORMAL PROJECT MANAGEMENT PROCESS

Because of the complexity in creating change and setting up trauma support systems, organizations should use a formal project management process. If an organization has never used this, it may be seen as excruciatingly detailed and tedious. But having a solid approach will result in a successful project. Every time there is a need to change direction, or drop a proposal from the project, or initiate a new proposal, or where there is a failure to meet a deadline, these actions can be defended as a result of the formal project management process.

There are several tools that are used in this process and they include: a charter, a reporting assignment matrix, and a to-do list and schedule. These elements are crucial to the project's success.

Charter: The charter defines the parameters in which project work will take place.

> The charter [outlines] the purpose, goals and objectives of the project, along with the critical success factors, strategy, interim and end products, scope, schedule, budget, constraints, planning

assumptions, risk assessment, project organizational impacts, reporting relationships, project priority, sponsor responsibilities, completion criteria and the project charter approvals. Ultimately, these approvals are absolutely crucial for [the lead, as the lead will have a document that details what is expected of him or her, their committee and who is on board for support.][1]

Reporting Assignment Matrix: This matrix is also known as the RAM, another tool within the formal project management process. Essentially, no matter at what stage the project develops, the lead and the Action Committee members

> ... always [decide] first who [has] to approve each stage of the work. The lower down [the chain of command] the reporting level the faster the work [gets approved and is acted on]. The higher up [the chain of command] the reporting level [is], the more likely there [could] be a delay.[2]

The To-Do List and the Schedule: At the start of each week, the lead should "review the to-do list and the schedule to [ascertain] what [is] expected to be accomplished in the coming week, by whom and who else would be impacted by the work either being completed or late."[3] The items on the to-do lists will help the lead plan the week. These two tools are the most important action tools at the lead's disposal.

KEY #4—ASSESSING THE ORGANIZATIONAL NEED FOR TRAUMA SUPPORT SYSTEMS

People realize that there is immense value in sharing similar experiences, especially ones that have resulted in trauma for an individual. As a result, peer support has existed in informal ways in families, in organizations and in communities for as long as people have lived together in groups.

There are some organizations where employees know who the peer supporters are and do indeed reach out to them in times of need. Often, the organization itself is not aware that these actions are happening or that these informal groups exist.

On the positive side, peers are a valuable asset when needed. On the negative side, many of these informal peers, though sincere in their desire to help, have not all reached positive growth themselves. Nor have they been formally trained to provide safe support for those in need.

The need for formal trauma support systems, which may include the informal peer support that already exists, validates undergoing an assessment of the organizational infrastructure to help employees address good mental health and safety in the workplace. The organizational assessment needs to be done using the many practices, resources and information that are available today, often for free. The results can be cost-effective and ensure buy-in from members or employees, when the organization is being proactive in implementing measures and supports to ensure a mentally healthy work environment. (*See* chapter 2 for tools on assessing the organization's awareness.)

There is new information being released monthly to substantiate the financial and economical value, and the need for good mental health practices and policies in the organization. If the only support is that of an informal peer group, known only among a few employees, then chances are the organization needs to move toward establishing an additional formal system. If the organization does not act responsibly, it may be forced to do so through provincial legislation. Where change is forced or legislated for organizations, the change is never as successful.

KEY #5—ESTABLISHING THE BUSINESS CASE

Any major operational changes within the organization can cause worry, unease and anxiety among the employees. It is therefore important to develop a business case for creating change in the workplace.

"Essentially, a business case is a strategic plan that takes advantage of an opportunity to create change. . . . [and] there is a basic flow to how a business case rolls out."[4] There are five essential phases that need to be followed in presenting the business case. These are:

1. [Establish] the case for change that clearly defines the need for the investment. . . .
2. [Acquire] a wide range of change options to achieve the goals defined in the first phase.
3. . . . [Analyze] these options to see which can be achieved and which are the best options to meet the established goals. . . .
4. [Make] recommendations that can be initiated to the goals.
5. . . . Manage and evaluate the changes.[5]

Guarding Minds @ Work is an excellent resource to help develop the business case. (*See* chapter 2, p. 14.)

KEY #6—RESEARCHING BEST PRACTICES

When it comes to researching best practices, the key is to determine if these practices really are the best ones and not just statements of claim that the organization is making. Where organizations claim to have excellent processes in place, it is imperative to talk to the boots on the ground to ensure these processes actually exist, that they are being used and are helpful. If employees are not taking advantage of the services being offered to them, then this is probably not a best practice but merely an attempt to alleviate organizational guilt by appearing to be doing something.

Once organizations with best practices have been identified, it is then necessary to beg, borrow or buy as many of their ideas as possible. Every organization that is doing this kind of work is the type that wants to help others. Generally, they are willing to share their ideas and techniques, as well as the lessons they have learned. However, no matter what is shared by other organizations, it is essential that trauma support systems are developed to fit and suit specific organizational needs. Other organizations' ideas and approaches can be used to guide the development but there is no such thing as a "cookie-cutter" approach in setting up a trauma support system.

KEY #7—DETERMINING THE LANGUAGE TO BE USED

In order to create change, organizations need consistency, that is, using and understanding the same language to address the issues that are happening in its workplace. There must be efforts to communicate the meaning behind the words used. The Action Committee must ensure that everyone understands and is using definitions in the same way for trauma within the workplace, for operational stress injuries, for post-traumatic stress, compassion fatigue, vicarious trauma and moral injury. Everyone must clearly understand how these injuries can occur and should know what the signs and symptoms might look like.

KEY #8—CREATING A COMMUNICATIONS STRATEGY

When any process is about organizational change, this means that everyone working for the organization will be affected. Therefore, everyone has to be involved in one way or another, even if that involvement is as simple as receiving ongoing communication about the program.

Communications is often underrated in terms of its impact on an organization's ability to move forward. There is also the tendency to hold back information until everything is working fine. But members or staff need to be informed at each step that is taken to implement change. This will ensure that everyone will have confidence in the organization's ability to move this process along.

The following tips are offered on how to use communications to the best advantage of both the Action Committee and the organization's members or staff.

Tip #1: Be Aware of the 15-70-15 Rule

Depending on the size of the organization, the 15-70-15 rule may or may not be a factor to consider (*see* illustration 3.1).... for those who need it, what this rule means is that [the committee] will generally find that there are fifteen percent of the people [in the organization] who will support—almost unequivocally—the objectives and benefits of [mental health and safety within the workplace]. This group is already convinced that what is about to start is something that should have been done already. At the other end, [most] will find fifteen percent in the organization .. will never accept [mental health in the workplace] as having any merit or value.

In between, [there is] seventy percent of the workforce just waiting to be convinced or informed about the value of [good mental health and safety within the workplace. The committee should] take advantage of the opportunity to talk to this group as soon aspossible; they are waiting to hear [more. If the organization doesn't] follow up with them, they may become part of the fifteen percent who are negative about change. It is always easier to be dismissive about a project requiring change than it is to get involved and work with it. If [the wait] is too long, then the damage will have been done and it will be much harder to change people's attitudes.

Illustration 3.1: The 15 – 70 –15 Rule

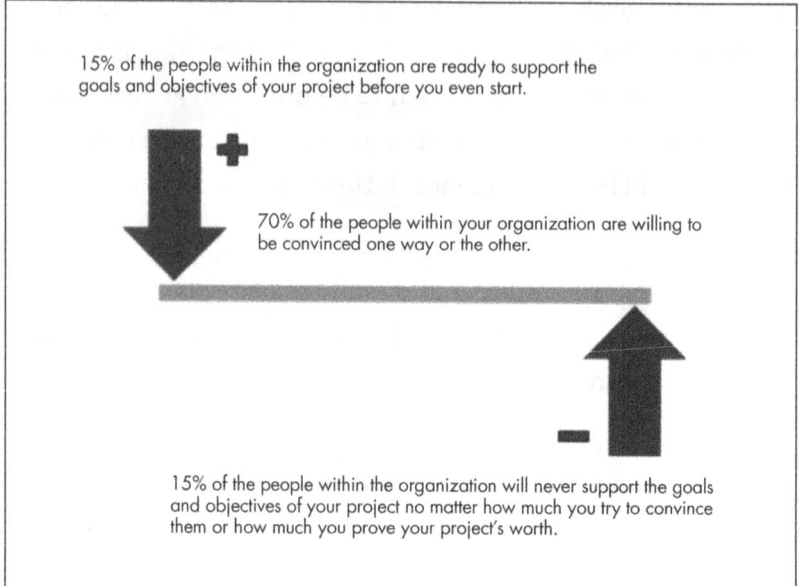

Tip #2: Don't Mislead People

Integrity is paramount when it comes to telling the truth about what [the Action Committee] is trying to accomplish. Some [people] believe that only the good news should be conveyed to employees. However, [many organizations have] discovered that they received the most support from the . . . staff when [they] revealed their weaknesses and mistakes, and [their] desire to address them now that they were acknowledged.

Tip #3: Make [Events] a Reason to Celebrate

[The committee should] announce every success . . ., no matter how small it may seem. [One of the authors, Syd Gravel,] met with the executive of [organization Y] to talk about why [organization X] was perceived as being so successful [in implementing cultural change,] when . . . [organization Y] wasn't, even though [it] had many more successful accomplishments than [organization X] did in the area of [cultural change].

What was revealed in discussions was that very few [people in organization Y] . . . knew about their work in the area of [creating change within the workplace,] since they didn't incorporate a communications strategy in their plan, which celebrated their successes. Therefore, it appeared . . . in their organization . . . that they had done very little, or nothing at all, to create the changes they needed. It's important [for the organization] to brag about itself]!

Tip #4: Use Your Own People to Support Your Communications Efforts

[The organization needs to] communicate comments from [its own] staff that show their support for the work being done. Nothing reinforces the efforts of an organizational change project as strongly as support at the grassroots level.

Tip #5: Answer Every Challenge Positively

As in every organization, the water-cooler gossip network [is] healthy. Every now and then, someone will start a negative rumour about the work [the Action Committee] is trying to accomplish. . . . Rumours start as a result of strongly held beliefs, which may be based on perception only. Yet, for many, perception is reality, so regardless of how offensive the rumour may be, there is usually a reason for it, which many believe validates their concerns.

If someone takes time to challenge [the intent of the] work, it is probably because they feel strongly enough about it to express their own thoughts and beliefs [and they have a lived experience that has validated their point of view.]

[The Action Committee] needs to take the time to respond to any rumours that are circulating in relation to the work being done. [The committee should] thank staff for expressing their concerns and provide facts about what [is being accomplished]. This helps to negate their concerns. [Well-crafted non-answers should never be used when trying to create a sincere change for the better within an organization.] People are fed up with this type of non-response and won't accept this kind of manipulation.

Tip #6: Share the Results with Others[6]

The Action Committee should share any results it has learned. There are many organizations looking for help in starting or improving their approach to trauma management and peer support. And not only successes but failings should also be shared. It is important to ensure that other organizations learn from mistakes made by others and don't repeat them.

KEY #9—DEVELOPING AND SUPPORTING ACCESSIBILITY TO RESOURCES

The Action Committee should create and provide a list of resources for the organization and ensure that it is accessible to everyone. The list should identify medical doctors with trauma awareness; trauma-certified psychiatrists, psychologists and psychotherapists; and mental health trauma therapists and social workers. Support groups, trauma-focused alternative care groups and other relevant resources should be listed and accessible to all members or employees as well.

It is important to look into the types of services that the organization's employee assistance program (EAP) offers compared to what the organization may need. In general, EAPs are not designed to address trauma-related issues. Their strength is in addressing stress in the workplace. But there is a significant difference between stress and trauma. When an employee is feeling "blue," most services under the EAP may provide what is required to help them get through this. However, when an employee is suffering the effects of depression, anxiety or trauma, much more help may be necessary. While the EAP provider may have these services, the organization may have to ask for them specifically to ensure employees have access when trauma occurs.

If there is a provincially funded workers compensation program to support members through injury or illness, then the organization needs a support mechanism in place to help employees navigate their way through the paperwork and bureaucracy. The last thing employees need, while they are suffering from a mental disorder, which lessens their ability to think and act to their full potential, is to deal with a complex bureaucracy on their own.

In some provinces, legislation has been passed in addressing PTSD for first responders that has reversed the onus for employees to prove their PTSD is a work-related injury. This legislation puts the onus on the employer to disprove it. However, more work has to be done so that other work-related injuries such as depression, compassion fatigue, vicarious trauma and anxiety are also included in the legislation.

KEY #10—ESTABLISHING A PROACTIVE APPROACH THROUGH TRAUMA SUPPORT SYSTEMS

There are several things that can be done by the Action Committee to encourage the organization to deal proactively with trauma-related work injuries.

One area that can be looked at is the reintegration of employees into the workplace. This is called the Mental Health Case Management process. It will satisfy the needs of both the organization to deal with an employee who is suffering from a mental illness or injury, as well as the employee's need to feel safe, secure and cared for in a respectful way in the workplace.

This management process is intended to enable an employee, or member, to return to work quickly, to regain their health over time in a productive manner with the assistance of managers skilled in working with those who have suffered mental illness or injury.

When a process such as this does not exist, individual employees, or members, decide on their own who will and who will not know about their need for help. It also leaves the decision about whom to trust and whom not to trust to the individual; this is usually based on their own personal experience with their peers and their supervisor, and their assessment of what to expect from both groups.

With no process in place, the onus is on managers to determine on their own how they will manage an employee who is known to them to be suffering from a mental illness or injury. The lack of accountability within a framework in which to work can lead to many end results on how the organization supports—or does not support—them. The outcome will depend on how caring, compassionate and capable each individual manager is in working with mentally ill or injured employees. This becomes a hit-and-miss process where some individuals believe they have been well supported by their supervisor, while others are left feeling abandoned, abused, mistreated and even slandered.

In developing Mental Health Case Management, there are two issues to be addressed:

1) How an employee is to be reintegrated into work and what support they receive is to be decided by the support team involved in the individual's case. No supervisor or manager would make this decision.

2) As a result of this clearly defined process, employees with a diagnosed mental illness or injury will know that their case will be managed by a team of concerned individuals who are working together to assist in their recovery and return to work.

The Mental Health Case Management process would also include representatives from human resources, health and wellness, and occupational health and safety, as well as middle managers, and an association/union representative.

This team of various representatives would be tasked with reviewing doctors' reports and considering their recommendations to determine if they can be carried out. The team would also have to consider what the injured or ill employee is willing to accept regarding restrictions on returning to work.

There has to be flexibility among all the parties in making a decision. Not all decisions will please either the injured/ill employee or management. The outcome, however, is to take the best decision possible that leads to the reintegration of the employee into the workplace. All decisions taken by the team should be considered final and only reviewable by the team as a whole, when and if circumstances change.

Finally, the Action Committee should look at and recommend:

> 1) The formation of a Mental Health Case Management Process and Team, which includes human resources, health and wellness, and occupational health and safety supervisors, as well as a representative from the union/association to help with the reintegration of employees.
>
> 2) The formation of a CISM Team which includes administrative support, communication protocols, and processes for the selection and training of its members.

3) The formation of Peer Support Systems by establishing a formal group, and considering the use of informal groups as well, which include administrative support, communication protocols and processes for the selection and training of its members.

4) The hiring or appointment of a Trauma Support Systems Lead as a full-time position.

5) The hiring or appointment of an Early Intervention Analyst as a full-time position.

6) The creation of Policies and Procedures for the organization to support all the previous recommendations.

7) The development of an early intervention system.

8) The development of family support.

An Action Committee that has followed all of the steps described in this chapter can be confident that it has done the necessary work to persuade the management of the organization of the benefits of establishing a trauma support system for its employees. By dealing with the ten key issues identified here, the committee should be in a healthy position to make recommendations to management that can be adopted by the organization.

4

Organizational Pre-Hiring Preparedness

For those organizations where the exposure to trauma-related injury is the greatest, that is, first responder services or agencies, they may want to consider how to prepare both applicants and candidates at the pre-hiring stage for positions in their organizations. There is also an opportunity to provide further education when the candidate is newly hired.

In his book *How to Survive PTSD and Build Peer Support*, Syd Gravel describes how not knowing what to be ready for led to far more damage occurring to him on the job than should have.

> Up until I experienced those fifty-six seconds, I had thought of myself as a fairly stable guy, with some great street sense and a solid character, who was able to work through any trauma that I saw or experienced as a police officer and as I thought I was expected to. . . .
>
> . . . In understanding what happens when trauma affects you, ignorance is certainly not bliss. In fact, it can slow down the healing process substantially. I have subsequently found out that there was very little about . . . the event itself, that was the problem for me. It was more about the inner workings of my mind in reaction to the event that had become the problem. . . .
>
> Since the late 1990s psychiatrists and psychologists now know much more about what is happening to the body and the mind, and how to address them in relation to reactions to trauma.

> Knowledge is power. In this case, knowledge about what is happening to you can help keep you healthy and alive. Having knowledge in advance about what can happen is absolutely precious. And I highly recommend that anyone working in [first responder] services educate themselves as to what could happen to them when reacting to trauma.
>
> I wish I had known about the effects of trauma and PTSD, and its impact on the body and mind, and what can help to begin the healing process. By knowing all this and being able to address my reactions when they happened, I probably would never have become a victim of PTSD.[1]

At the Pre-Hiring Stage

The authors suggest that there is a need to invest in resilience training for first responders and military before they begin their careers. They also believe that this need goes well beyond these groups. Such training should include any organization, service or group that deals with day-to-day human tragedy. This would include social workers dealing with those in community housing or with children, or with society's poor and homeless; emergency department doctors and nurses; security personnel; trauma therapists; teachers and church leaders. Frontline responders can encompass civilians from all walks of life where trauma can occur on a daily basis—not just for police officers, firemen, paramedics and other frontline personnel.

Opportunities to educate the next generation of potential candidates can be found at the community college and university level. In fact, this is the first step that the organization can take to discuss psychological health and safety issues at the pre-hire stage. Both authors have presented information several times over the years to both police foundations and to students pursuing health and wellness careers at numerous provincial colleges. The students are always very attentive and interested. The authors were able to convey to them the need for self-care and peer support, as well as discuss with them the consequences of prolonged trauma exposure. They have been able to show, through their lived experiences with traumatic events, that individuals can survive, thrive, endure and still pursue a rewarding career.

The authors also ensured that there was a discussion about preparing mentally for a career on the front lines in first responder services by building resiliency which they will need in their future. Speaking to students or recruits early in their education can also open up a discussion on the stigma associated with mental illness. Organizations and recruiters can advise how important it is to take care of one's own mental health. Doing so in today's organizations is a strength and not a weakness. It is a positive step that starts with entry-level members or employees.

There is a significant opportunity for many organizations to reach out to potential job applicants and those candidates, who have already reached the pre-hiring phase, to prepare them for the psychological impacts of trauma over an extended period of time. Organizations need to begin at the earliest possible time in their potential new hires to prepare them for the job.

On Being Hired

There is a new generation moving into the front lines of first responder organizations. They are smart, healthy, knowledgeable and family-oriented, and they are very much in tune with their own needs. They use many communication tools that provide them with considerable information. This makes the task of mental preparedness much easier as this generation will be eager for information that will prepare them for the trauma exposures and conflict they will have to endure on the job of their chosen profession.

This should also provide opportunities for first responder organizations and agencies to implement policies and procedures that provide both a physically and mentally safe and secure work environment for this new workforce. Organizations can use many of the resources and tools that are now available (e.g., the mental health standards for workplaces) to educate young recruits or potential candidates for hire at the start of their careers.

Gone are the days—or they should be—when young officers or other first responders are baptized by fire, with young rookies sent to view a violent crime scene to toughen them up or young paramedics joining their organizations without ever having seen a dead body. Studies have shown that younger police officers with less experience are at an increased risk to develop PTSD symptoms following a traumatic event. This is likely due to the fact that they have not yet developed sufficient coping strategies to deal with the high level of stress associated with police work or with the ongoing exposures to trauma that they are repeatedly subjected to.[2]

Today, there is also much more known about the development of the brain. The adult brain is not fully developed until age twenty-two or three. When rookies were hired as cadets, police services were really sending adolescents into the line of fire. They were setting the stage for a career that, at some point, would potentially include

PTSD, well before these young brains could handle the trauma to which they are exposed.

First responder services need to safeguard young recruits and other young recently hired employees. More than ever, organizations are obliged not to send their workforce into psychological harm's way. Unfortunately, frontline responder organizations are in the business of doing just exactly that. So, at the very least, these services need to prepare their workforces for the consequences of repeated exposure to traumatic events as a result of being sent into potentially harmful situations over and over again. The earlier that future prospects are prepared and learn about good mental health, the better for both them and the employer.

Organizations also need to make certain that their young recruits are psychologically healthy to do the job. Most leading-edge organizations are taking their candidates through psychological testing and clinical interviews. There are particularly good tests to determine previous trauma exposure. They can also learn if previous exposure has been processed and the candidate is healthy enough for the position.

When the recruiting process is completed and the new recruit first reports, this provides another opportunity for the organization to provide additional information on the strategies, and policies and procedures, that are in place to create a mentally healthy work environment. These new members are fresh, eager and energetic; naïve and impressionable; and intelligent and innovative. Because they are eager to fit in, they will be looking for what is "the norm" on how to think, behave and survive in their new environment. This is the ideal time to give them the best tools to deal with their new job.

The organization needs to make certain that there is no possibility of them jumping onto the "stigma bandwagon" around mental illness. Now is the time to show that the organization supports all efforts to encourage its members to seek help, when and if it is needed, both for a physical and a mental injury or illness. First impressions are significant at this stage. Someone with a lived experience as a peer supporter can also speak to young recruits. They can share with them how the stigma of mental illness can hamper a member's recovery from a significant trauma.

This person can let them know that there is a trusted peer support system in place not only for them but also for their family. The peer can discuss what resources are available to them in case they need them. It is also important to advise new recruits that they may never need these supports but they are there if they do. And these young recruits need to be reminded that, if their colleague has a mental health challenge, it is their responsibility to do what they can to support them—without judgment—and engage the peer support system to help.

There are several opportunities for an organization to reach out to potential candidates at the pre-hiring stage. Once the new recruit (or employee) joins the organization, this provides another chance to discuss mental health and its importance in dealing with the traumas that new hires may experience in doing their job.

5

Organizational Support for Families

As new members—or recruits—come through the door of an organization for the first time, so does their family. For first responder services or agencies, there are two questions that need to be addressed: 1) Why is it important for an organization to educate families about the nature of the job their loved one is about to take on? 2) What information and resources does it have in place to support a family when their loved one suffers a trauma-induced injury from the job?

Failing the Family

Syd Gravel provides a classic example of an organization's response to his family's appeal for help from his employer, when he suffered on-the-job trauma and the effects of PTSD as a consequence. By not knowing what to do—or even if it should be doing something—the organization did considerable harm to him and his family, and it took a long time before the family unit trusted the management of the police service involved.

> At 0500 hours on Sunday, Judy Gravel received a call from the police service informing her that her husband had been involved in a shooting. She was told that he was fine. But he had requested that she be called to see

if she could come to the station. She had two young children—ages four and five—in her care and it was very early Sunday morning. She needed to find a babysitter if she was to go to the station. She reached out to her friends and neighbours to find someone who would help.

An unmarked police car arrived to drive her to the station, which was a forty-five minute journey from her home. The two undercover officers had no information about the incident her husband was involved in. In fact, they didn't even know his health status. They had only been asked to drive her to the station. So, for forty-five minutes, she rode in the back of the car with no information to prepare her for what was coming.

She arrived at the station and was met by a lawyer that the police association had hired to represent her husband. The lawyer informed her that she had nothing to worry about, that his rights were being protected. From what, she wondered?

She was then seated in the cafeteria to wait until she could see her husband. As she sat there, another shift was coming in to work. The officers were seated at tables all around her discussing what they had heard about the incident her husband was involved in. It wasn't until one of the officers recognized her that everyone was told to shut up and keep their opinions to themselves. But by then the damage had been done. She was starting to have panic attacks and her mind was racing with all kinds of questions, Is he going to lose his job? Is he facing criminal charges? How will we live without an income? Will I lose him?

Organizational Support for Families

After several hours, her husband arrived with the lawyer. Judy was told to take him home for now. Because he had been told by so many people not to talk until such time as the case was properly investigated, he refused to speak to her about what happened during the drive home. Not being able to speak about the incident, they spoke of nothing at all.

When they arrived home, he started to have panic and anxiety attacks right away. He became hypervigilant and overreacted to every little thing Judy said or did. She was afraid to move an inch for fear of triggering an over-the-top reaction from him. Finally, he fell asleep but only after several very difficult hours.

From this point things only got worse. After several days, Judy asked her husband to get some help; he refused. He didn't think there was anything wrong with him that time could not heal.

After several months, during which he was exhibiting some very unhealthy behaviours, Judy had reached the point where she simply wanted him to get help. His behaviour was no longer that of the man she loved and had married.

Judy called the police station for help. The officer who answered the call listened as she described her husband's behaviour. The officer asked, "What platoon is he with?"

"E-Platoon," she said.

"Well, they work in three days. Call back then to speak to his staff," he responded and hung up on her.

She called the police association next and they transferred her to the president. He listened carefully and advised he didn't know what could be offered. But he said he would find out. He called back shortly after to say they had found a psychologist who worked with soldiers returning from Vietnam. The psychologist was willing to speak to her husband.

Judy reached out to the doctor and booked a meeting. She then offered her husband a choice: a visit to the doctor or else. He chose the visit to the doctor. When they arrived at the office, Judy walked up to the doctor, looked him squarely in the face and said, "This is my husband, I need you to fix him!" She then turned to her husband and said, "Work with the doctor to get yourself fixed!" Then she told them both that she would be seated outside until they were done.

From that first visit onward, Syd and the doctor got along famously. And the rest is history.

They made it through all right but not without a lot of damage being done to both during the early days of the event and for many years afterward as a result of the trauma suffered by both Syd and his family.

It makes no sense whatsoever that first responder organizations will send their members into harm's way because of the nature of the job but fail, as an employer, to educate the families of their employees about the potential risks of work-related trauma from the job.

When mental health issues surface in an organization's members, it is the family that is the first to notice them. Families need to know what to do and where to go for help. Logically, the first contact should be the organization for whom their family member works.

What the Organization Can Do

PRE-HIRING STAGE

The first opportunity for an organization to speak to the family is at the recruitment or pre-hire stage. In fact, throughout the hiring process, there are many opportunities to interact with both the member and their family.

The organization can arrange for a psychological interview not only for the potential recruit but also for their family. This is an opportunity for a mental health professional to talk about the candidate's mental health and resiliency both for them and their family. Home interviews can also be conducted through a veteran member or a retiree on contract. The seasoned member/interviewer can discuss with the family unit how they can be impacted by this new career and how to mitigate the challenges they will face. The family will learn about what measures the organization has in place such as peer support and a health benefits package that provides assistance to both the member and the entire family. Should the candidate be successful, they and their family will have the support they need.

ORIENTATION STAGE

Once a candidate is identified to become a member of the organization, there are usually several weeks of in-house orientation. This is an ideal opportunity for further education for the family as well. The orientation organizers can dedicate a day or an evening for the mandatory dissemination of information to the family about the resources and benefits available should they need to reach out.

The family needs to know that there may be times when their loved one will experience calls that are abnormal or traumatic but that they can handle it because of their training and education. The family must be reassured that, when their loved one does encounter something that will jeopardize their ability to cope, the organization will help both them and their loved one through it.

This is a chance for an organization to identify for family members, as well as the recruit, the signs, symptoms and normal reactions to the abnormal traumatic exposures they may experience. More often than not, it is the family who first notices a change in behaviour.

The organization can provide information about what services and resources are available to deal with PTSD and other mental health challenges. It can hand out information on the health benefit plan and what it covers, or if there is an employer assistance program (EAP) in place, and advise that it has invested in and set up a peer support team that the family can call on when needed. Any information package that is handed out should include information on how to contact the peer support team. (The organization may want to keep in mind that some family members could be recruited as peer supporters. *See* chapter 9, p. 97.) At the welcoming or badge ceremony, the chief or CEO can reaffirm that the organization will support members and their families as they start their career. This orientation period may be the only time that there is an opportunity to address the family on the topic of wellness and what the service is doing to create and maintain a healthy workplace.

The Importance of a Family Relationship

The authors have made frequent references throughout the book about the importance of a family to employees and to the organization in which they work. If employees, or members, have a solid family relationship, they will be happier and healthier than those who do not have such support.

There are studies that have proved that people who have strong, healthy family support systems are themselves healthier and long-lived. Dr. Robert Waldinger, a psychiatrist and psychoanalyst at Harvard Medical Center is the director of the longest study on happiness. The Harvard Study of Adult Development was conducted over a period of seventy-five years.[1] Out of 724 men, 60 are still alive and in their 90s.

The bottom line of this study was the discovery that "good relationships keep us happier and healthier." The study was broken down into three categories:

1. Social connections are really good for us. Isolation kills. Isolation is toxic and results in less happiness and health. One in five people are believed to be lonely.
2. It is not the number of friends we have, but the quality of those relationships that matter. Living in an environment of a high conflict marriage with little or no affection is very bad for your health. Warm relationships are protective. Those who were most satisfied in their relationship at age 50 were healthiest at age 80.
3. Good relationships don't just protect our bodies; they protect our brains. As people transition from work to retirement, it is best to replace their workmates with playmates.[2]

When Dr Waldinger talks about relationships, he means the connection with family, friends and community.

Family relationships do not mean that a person has to be married or in a significant full-time intimate relationship. People can have meaningful and powerful connections with other family members and long-time close friends. The two authors are good examples of where their connections played a significant role in their survival and health. Yet their support structures were different.

Syd believes and tells everyone that, if it were not for his wife Judy, to whom he has been married for forty years, he would not be here today. As a family member, Judy knew what to do when she realized that he was no longer able to cope with his PTSD and had decided to take his life. She took the bold step to ask for help from the Ottawa Police Service. Whenever one sees Syd, it will not be hard to find Judy. They are a connected, loving couple, with children and grandchildren and the envy of many who will never have or experience the depth of their relationship.

Brad was married for twenty-one years and is the father of two successful daughters. When he divorced, he maintained a professional and respectful relationship with his former wife and her family. His strength comes from the connection he has with his daughters, his parents, his sister and, most significantly, his brother Bruce. Brad's strength also comes from his many strong friendships that he has maintained for decades. These long-term, loyal, trusted and meaningful relationships provided him with protection and support. Brad's immediate family has survived trauma exposure, child abuse, terminal illness and addiction. Brad's circle of family and friends has kept him strong and resilient.

To a degree, there has always been some connection between a person's work and family. But, historically, organizations have limited connections to annual children's Christmas parties and dances, and maybe a summer picnic.

Leading-edge organizations that are serious about creating mentally healthy workplaces will maintain ongoing communication with both their employees and their families. They may provide weekly publications that celebrate their organization, describe success stories or that feature charitable initiatives and fundraisers. Information can be sent out electronically, posted to a website or communicated through any number of social media. The idea is to maintain a connection to the family and to assure them that the organization also cares for their well-being.

Building a partnership with the family may be the key to supporting their loved one as they recover from a trauma or work-related injury. Strong family relationships are essential in the recovery of an organization's employees from work-related trauma or a mental injury.

6

Middle Management Leadership

One of the key levels in an organization is middle management.[1] In many ways, middle managers are the glue that holds an organization together. Or they should be. Middle management is in a unique position to take a leadership role in helping the organization implement mental health strategies and in developing peer support teams.[2]

Building Trust

Middle managers occupy a position in the organization between frontline staff, or members, and senior management. They can be a filter for both groups. They can also be detrimental to an organization that is trying to implement change through negative thinking or failing to relay information about what is happening at the senior level or how the frontline is reacting to change. Too often middle managers hide in their office with the door closed. They need to connect with the frontline staff as much as possible.

Middle managers need to be resilient and trustworthy for both senior management and the front lines. They need to be visible, approachable and open-minded. They often are required to act as a filter between the two levels of the organization, removing negativity and toxicity but, at the same time, ensuring that both sides receive clear and unbiased information.

One of the best ways for middle managers to build trust with the workforce is to show support by attending social functions to which their members have invited them. They should be present at pre-shift briefings or the parade or take part in ride-a-longs whenever possible. This is not an invitation for middle management to become overly familiar with those they supervise. In fact, a smart middle manager will attend an event early, speak to as many employees and family members as possible, consume no or minimal alcohol and leave early.

The responsibility to create a workplace environment of trust among management levels puts significant stress and pressure on middle managers. They are often alone with no one to talk to. Yet they are expected to be the open-minded communicators reporting issues between senior management and the workforce; watching for signs of work-related trauma, stress and anxiety; and ensuring that there is a way to encourage employees to seek assistance and support, when they encounter mental health challenges.

Training Middle Managers

Once an organization has decided to implement strategies and measures to create a mentally healthy workplace and, along with this goal, to provide assistance to its employees through a peer support program, middle managers will play a major role, particularly in early intervention.

Middle managers have a responsibility and a duty to care for the employees under their supervision. They have a duty to keep the workforce as safe as possible under all circumstances. They need to identify and address early behaviours that impact the performance of staff and the overall team dynamics of shift work.

Middle managers require the tools to understand how to manage stress, how to recognize the signs of work-related trauma and how to provide support to their staff. It is for this reason that middle managers need to learn about mental health issues and how to overcome the stigma of mental illness among employees, so that they can ensure that individuals are comfortable in seeking assistance and support from the organization.

Middle managers must also be trained to look for behaviours that may be an indication of a work-related trauma, or some other issue the individual is dealing with. Middle management must be particularly alert to the risk factors in first responder services that can create work-related traumas.

Most often coworkers will advise about a change in their colleague's behaviour. This is a first warning to middle management that follow-up is required. A first step is to seek information from the records management system. This includes looking for details that could indicate the individual is being exposed to more trauma than they are able to handle (e.g., attendance at a high number of death calls [*see* chapter 11, p. 118 for more information]).

Changes in behaviour in individuals are usually indicators that they are facing some mental health changes.[3] Or they may be dealing with a family crisis that is overwhelming and causing on-the-job issues. Addressing these behaviours at an early stage allows for a number of positive opportunities. If middle managers have met the individual's family, they may feel comfortable in reaching out to them to inquire if there is any support that can be provided at home as well.

Effective Tools for Middle Management

PROJECT SAFEGUARD

One tool that may be useful to middle management is Project Safeguard. This program was originally set up to protect investigators in Internet child exploitation units; these members were identified as being at a higher risk to experience secondary traumatic stress because of the nature of the investigations and their repeated exposure.

Most leading-edge police services use it to protect members who investigate fatal motor vehicle collisions, homicides and child abuse, as well as for covert operators and forensic death scene investigators.

This program involves psychological screening, including a test and an interview by a qualified practitioner. It also involves a level of mental preparation and ongoing monitoring. Much of the responsibility rests with the supervisor or middle manager who will mentally prepare and monitor those in high-risk positions. The term *safeguarding your members* refers to this program and how an organization ensures that the member is healthy for a high-risk position and that measures are in place to maintain their health.

ROAD TO MENTAL READINESS (R2MR)

Another tool that may be useful to middle managers is the Road to Mental Readiness or R2MR. It was developed by the Department of National Defence (DND). Its "goal . . . is to improve short-term performance and long-term mental health outcomes"[4] for the Canadian Armed Forces. It is based on the concept of resilience, which "is the capacity to recover quickly from a trauma."[5]

The training program was adapted by the Mental Health Commission of Canada, in partnership with DND and the Calgary Police Services, "to fit a police organization's culture and values."[6] This training tool focuses on teaching mental resilience and reducing the stigma associated with mental illness. R2MR is specially designed for supervisors and middle managers to teach them 1) how to support a healthy working environment within their unit, 2) how to recognize the signs of mental illness and 3) how to address members who show signs of needing support. Middle managers also learn how to maintain resilience themselves. (In 2014, York Regional Police brought the training to Ontario.)

The purpose of this training tool is to bring awareness to middle managers responsible for supervising police officers who operate in high-risk positions where they are at considerable risk of encountering an operational stress injury. Today, leading-edge organizations ensure that all supervisors and middle managers receive R2MR training. The Ontario Police College has mandated that every new provincial constable be provided with this training. York Regional Police have their own trainers and have committed to delivering the program to every member of their service. In 2016, R2MR is also being introduced to fire and paramedic services.

Suicide Awareness

Available statistics indicate that "more than twice as many peace officers die because of suicide than are killed in the line of duty."[7] What is important for middle managers to know is that "eighty percent of people who attempt suicide tell somebody first via their actions or actual statements."[8] Middle managers must know what to do when they learn that a member of the organization is showing signs of suicide ideation. It is important that middle management keeps the lines of communication open, so that employees are comfortable coming to them about suicidal indications in a colleague. Early intervention strategies can be developed to help identify more than eighty percent of those who talk about or are at risk to attempt suicide. Policies and procedures must state clearly to notify a supervisor or manager if a member is suicidal.

The problem is that most supervisors don't know what to do or say. They have little or no training around the issues of suicide or how to be comfortable in dealing with it. When they do try to intervene, it is often a very quick and uncomfortable conversation. There is a training tool for middle managers and supervisors called safeTALK, developed by LivingWorks, a leader in suicide intervention training. safeTALK is described as follows:

> safeTALK is a half-day alertness training that prepares anyone over the age of 15, regardless of prior experience or training, to become a suicide-alert helper. Most people with thoughts of suicide don't truly want to die, but are struggling with the pain in their lives. Through their words and actions, they invite help to stay alive. safeTALK-trained helpers can recognize these invitations and take action by connecting them with life-saving intervention resources, such as caregivers trained in ASIST.
>
> Since its development in 2006, safeTALK has been used in over 20 countries around the world, and more than 200 selectable video vignettes have been produced to tailor the program's audio-visual component for diverse audiences. safeTALK-trained helpers are an important part of suicide-safer communities, working alongside intervention resources to identify and avert suicide risks.[9]

ASIST is also a training program for supervisors that develops skills to enable them to identify the risk factors for suicide. The training enables them to become more comfortable in communicating with an individual and in providing quality intervention options. If the organization has a peer support system in place, the supervisor can team up with a trained peer. The supervisor will be responsible for developing a plan and recommending or providing professional mental health resources. (*See* chapter 10, p. 103 for more information about ASIST and other workshops for suicide intervention training.)

An organization that is serious about providing an all-round healthy workplace will need the help of its middle management group to buy into the concept. In doing so, organizations need to offer and support all types of training for these managers. After all, middle management is the key link to move the organization forward to support mental health.

7

Developing a Critical Incident Stress Management (CISM) Team

Many organizations will set up a Critical Incident Stress Management (CISM) Team before creating a peer support team. In larger more structured organizations, there can be some value in keeping the CISM and Peer Teams separate. This is not to say that the Peer Support Team is less important. In most cases, however, it is better to blend the responsibilities and have peer support members trained and experienced in both general peer support and CISM.

CISM is a set of tools designed mainly for trauma exposure intervention. As such, the development of this team has always been viewed as a priority in first responder organizations because of the trauma exposures faced regularly by their members.

The CISM Model

The pioneering organization for the CISM model is the International Critical Incident Stress Foundation (ICISF). The original intervention model was called the Mitchell Model after Dr. Jeffrey T. Mitchell who developed it in the early 1980s. It is now known as the ICISF Model and is used worldwide as the guideline for trauma response and management in first responder services such as police, fire and paramedics. CISM is a comprehensive intervention system.

There are seven core components of CISM. Each of these is unique to the needs of the trauma event and the organization itself. Whatever the crisis, there will be a method that fits and that can be applied to an individual, a small group, a family or across the organization. The components are:

> 1. Pre-crisis preparation. This includes stress management education, stress resistance, and crisis mitigation training for both individuals and organizations.
>
> 2. Disaster or large-scale incident, as well as school and community support programs including demobilizations, informal briefings, "town meetings" and staff advisement.
>
> 3. Defusing. This is a 3-phase, structured, small group discussion provided within hours of a crisis for purposes of assessment, triaging, and acute symptom mitigation.
>
> 4. Critical Incident Stress Debriefing (CISD) refers to the "Mitchell Model" 7-phase, structured group discussion, usually provided 1 to 10 days post crisis, and designed to mitigate acute symptoms, assess the need for follow-up and, if possible, provide a sense of post-crisis psychological closure.
>
> 5. One-on-one crisis intervention/counseling or psychological support throughout the full range of the crisis spectrum.
>
> 6. Family crisis intervention, as well as organizational consultation.
>
> 7. Follow-up and referral mechanisms for assessment and treatment, if necessary.[1]

Much of the focus of the ICISF Model is working with groups. Applied properly and appropriately, the group debriefing system can be very productive. The reason is that, when a group is exposed to a traumatic event together, there is a bond due to the common ground of the experience. Some in the group may be traumatized more than others. In a debriefing, there is a natural tendency to bond, care for, validate and support each other in the group, especially those who are struggling. Those who are struggling realize they are not alone or isolated and they care for each other, often well after the debriefing is concluded.

There has been some controversy concerning these group debriefings.[2] But there is more supporting evidence that shows these debriefing sessions are helpful. The ICISF Model, in many cases, supports group work and is beneficial to a multidisciplinary team. It naturally supports the evolution of the group.

Developing a CISM Team

To develop a credible and trusted CISM Team, the organization needs to follow the same process as it would use in developing a peer support team. (*See* chapter 8.) All structured peer teams should consist of those with a lived experience of trauma exposure who are currently healthy and in positive growth. There should also be clinical direction from a mental health professional who has significant credentials in trauma response, intervention and therapy.

MENTAL HEALTH PROFESSIONALS AND CISM

The difference between CISM and peer support is that CISM requires more mental health trauma professionals. In the CISM model, a mental health professional needs to be present to lead and provide clinical direction during debriefing sessions. Some CISM teams are fortunate enough to have mental health professionals who volunteer their time to the team. Other CISM Teams utilize mental health professionals who are under contract. But no matter which structure the organization selects, mental health professionals must be available to the team.

These professionals must be capable of providing the service, understand the common character traits of the organization's members, and the idiosyncrasies of the service, and must be trusted by the members. The organization should not use the mental health professional, who provides direction and advice on discipline matters, or on any work-related matter, for the Human Resources Department.

To gain credibility and trust among the organization's members or staff, the mental health professional should interact with the members wherever possible. There are opportunities at pre-shift briefings for the mental health professional to be introduced and engaged. Many first responder organizations may also offer ride-a-longs for these professionals.

The Multidisciplinary CISM Team

The organization may want to consider developing a multidisciplinary CISM Team. For example, the York Region CISM Team currently has over fifty members. When this team was created in 1996, it was set up to serve police, fire, EMS, hospital emergency department staff, and the communicators and dispatchers for these groups. However, this type of team is rare.

The benefits of the multidisciplinary team have been outstanding because of the group work that engages all emergency service personnel impacted by the same trauma. It is extremely helpful for healing and processing the event, when there are people within the group who can fill in the blanks for others. And the natural tendency to support each other extends outside the borders of one organization.

Despite the differences between frontline services, there is a significant level of trust and respect due to the commonality of the roles in protecting and serving the community. Having a cross-section of frontline responders, who were "hands on" during the incident, provides a clear picture to the participants and an expanded nonjudgmental support network beyond a single service.

A multidisciplinary team also enables the organization to facilitate group interventions that are all-encompassing, that is, that include representatives from each of the responding organizations during the event. Along with police, fire and emergency services, representatives can be invited from court security, the coroner's office, crown prosecutors, private security, lifeguards, tow truck operators, body removal service, children's aid workers, volunteer search organizations and more. The purpose of a properly functioning CISM team is to ensure that the entire responding entity is taken care of.

CISM is designed to support caregivers. Although it would be rare to include a tow truck operator or lifeguard in a debriefing with frontline responders, it would be appropriate to reach out and ensure they have resources to assist and support them after a trauma exposure.

CHAPLAINS

It is important to consider using chaplains on the CISM Team. Many first responder organizations and hospitals have a chaplain program. Often they are utilized for ceremonies and special events but underutilized in the area of wellness and peer support. Their training and experience is relevant and transferrable in supporting those exposed to trauma. They support families and communities regularly as they deal with death and they have significant mental preparation and coping skills.

Chaplains in CISM are unique. They fall somewhere between the mental health professional's responsibilities and that of the peer supporter. They have a very important role to play because they are often trusted more than anyone else. In the military environment, the chaplain's office is visited often due to its open door policy. A chaplain on a CISM team or available in the system can be a valuable asset.

Deployment of the CISM Team

The benefit of having a CISM team trained under the ICISF Model is that the team can be deployed outside its jurisdiction. It can also be mixed and matched with other teams, which is similar to community response teams who trained under the National Organization for Victim Assistance (NOVA) Model.[3] Brad McKay co-led a team of CISM responders to New York City in 2002 to assist the Police Organization Providing Peer Assistance, known as POPPA, with interventions for NYPD officers who were adversely affected by 9/11. They showed up with three debriefing teams, each team with three peers and a mental health professional. They were surprised when they learned that they were going to be mixed and matched with other CISM-trained members from all over North America to do the debriefings.

Because of their common training, there were no complications and the interventions went well.

If the organization has a competent CISM team, the ICISF will coordinate requests for its assistance when disaster strikes. Several times in the U.S., CISM Teams have self-deployed and showed up wanting to help. What this does is throw needless confusion into an already complicated response process; it does more harm than good. There is a methodical system in place to provide assistance and direction will come through the ICISF or the Canadian Critical Incident Stress Foundation (CCISF).

Controversy and an Optional Approach

There has been some controversy on how the ICISF Model is managed and applied. The use of the Mitchell Model debriefing, without the presence of a mental health professional, can cause more harm than good. The Royal Ottawa Mental Health Centre's Operational Stress Injuries Clinic has collected evidence that suggests that an immediate psychological debriefing, using the CISM method without having a mental health professional present, is at best inept and at worst harmful.

Current best practices suggest that psychological first aid in most environments, where there is no mental health professional available, is the best way to focus on immediate needs. Psychological first aid will: 1) help an individual to feel connected, validated and safe; and 2) provide education about signs that may warrant seeking help. The idea is to "plant seeds" rather than initiate long-term contact.

An organization will find that using the ICISF Model will provide all the essential tools and training that members of the CISM Team will need. The model should be endorsed by the organization and team members need to be trained. (*See* chapter 10 on training.) But, if resources are lacking on the team in that a professional mental health worker cannot attend debriefings, then organizations should keep a debriefing at the psychological first aid and information level only.

This chapter has provided an overview of the steps that need to be taken for first responder organizations that have decided to set up a CISM team to provide trauma interventions for their members.

8

Developing Peer Support Teams

The authors have over fifty-five years of experience in the development and management of peer support teams. Since both their experiences with peer support are different, each of their perspectives and approaches are shared here.

Syd's work is entirely in informal peer support, which has been developed without any management involvement. It has been underground, secretive and hidden from the organization. He has never worked with a formal peer support program or worked outside of dealing with officers involved in fatal or near-fatal incidents. His is pure empathy work, with no formal training or psychological testing involved at the time.

Brad's work is both formal and informal, involves multiple services and is peer-driven. The peer support teams have been supported and endorsed by management, and members of the team are highly trained and include representatives from many first responder services.

Peer Support from Syd Gravel's Experience

Peer support is the foundation through which lived experience in positive growth connects with empathy for those who have been traumatized. Peer support provides help that is needed, whether it is medical or psychological, by directing the person to resources. It then supports the person seeking help through the healing process through reassurance and guidance. Once a person is strong enough, the peer support team lets them go without any obligation for the support that was offered.

Informal peer support has been in place for groups of people ever since humankind figured out the difference between empathy and sympathy. The value of speaking to someone who has survived a similar incident prior to one's own experience is invaluable in establishing a safe place for a survivor.

Syd believes that there are two fundamental requirements to work as a peer: 1) having empathy and 2) being in a positive growth stage.

Empathy is defined as "the action of understanding, being aware of, being sensitive to . . . feelings, thoughts, and experiences of another."[1] Empathy is about sharing a similar experience and understanding the pain and the suffering of someone else. Empathy is about having been there personally, having survived and being able to listen, understand and validate what another is experiencing.

A peer support person must also be in a positive growth stage. It is not good enough to simply have been a survivor. Unless the person is at a stage in their recovery, which is positive, they should not do the work required of a peer. It is essential that the person learns to live with their issues and recover before considering being a peer to someone else. As a part of a peer support team, each member will be viewed as an example of how to move forward. But, if that person has not yet fully recovered from their own lived experience, it is difficult to help someone else. Members of an informal peer support team must also know the difference between good and bad advice, and what the boundaries are in terms of providing support.

Far too many informal peers are willing to reach out to others who have lived a similar experience, based on the old adage that misery loves company. This belief is based on their own experience that nothing can be done to help oneself. There are also far too many informal peers who are justifiably bitter as a result of how they were, or are being, treated in their workplace. They have suffered what is known as sanctuary trauma, along with their work-related trauma.[2] Still dealing with their own issues of trust, particularly in the workplace, they should not be part of a peer support team themselves. They could do considerable damage to the newly injured.

The Legitimacy of Informal Peer Support

Syd believes that informal peer support is absolutely crucial for any organization or community, especially police services where his experiences were lived.

Police officers, among all first responders, are the only ones who have the legitimate authority and power to use a gun which can cause fatal injury. And, once used, they are immediately placed under investigation to determine if that use of force was legitimate, which at best can be determined as justified or, at worst, the officer can be charged with murder.

The officer, while going through the investigation, must also deal with the physical, psychological and emotional after-effects of the trauma that has been experienced. The last person they may want to speak to is a colleague or someone from the employee assistance program, who is part of a formal organizational structure. The injured officer is dealing with feelings of doubt and anger, and doesn't feel safe speaking to someone in the organization.

This is why having a group of empathetic informal peers to lean on is crucial. The members of this team will be in a positive growth position and they will have walked in similar situations. If this informal peer team is not part of the organization, it makes it easier for the person seeking support to open up and trust. However, it is important to note that, although the peer team may not be part of the organization, it doesn't mean that they don't understand how crucial their work is as peers and how careful they have to be not to do harm.

One of the most successful informal peer support groups in policing was established in Ottawa in 1988. The group was called Robin's Blue Circle. Seven "police officers got together, under the guidance of Dr. Pierre Turgeon, a professor at the University of Ottawa, to help each other through the effects of post-shooting trauma as a result of work-related incidents."[3]

There were several keys to the success of this informal peer support team.

1. They kept the group small so that there was comfort and safety in knowing who everyone else was and why they were there.
2. Initially, they included Dr. Turgeon as an integral part of their monthly meetings during the early stages. Eventually, as the peer team members gained strong positive growth on their own and began to understand the parameters in which they should work to offer support to each other, Dr. Turgeon was available only if required.

3. They established the purpose for meeting and set out rules and guidelines to meet their goal. The rules ensured that they focused on how they were feeling, letting each person speak openly without any interruptions.
4. They committed to watch over each other and to be there in times of need.
5. When bringing in a new person, they explained the rules and allowed that person time to speak and to share their experience when they were ready.

The original support group included "Robin Easey, a Nepean police officer with 21 Division, who survived a near-fatal bullet wound to the back of the head during a botched robbery."[4] The other original members included four officers who had been shot and had survived, and three members who had fatally shot a suspect. They

> saw the healing process as a circle back to their normal routine after having been involved in situations that had disrupted their daily life, thus, the name Robin's Blue Circle. Since 1988, the circle has grown to include police officers from across Canada. They understood each other as no one had ever understood them since their events.[5]

As of 2016, three of the founding members have died. Of the remaining four original members, only Syd continues to work as a peer and trauma support advisor.

This informal peer support group developed a philosophy about the type of support they needed to provide. They

> believe that officers involved in fatal or near-fatal incidents should not try to forget or pretend that the event never occurred [– denial of the events denies recovery]. They also

believe that officers should not stay alone, except when time alone is needed to gather their thoughts. What they need to know and learn is that the event is now part of their life and part of their character; they need to move on with their life and the knowledge of the incident entrenched within their life and who they are now. The process of accepting this is shown in the blue circle as seen in illustration 8.1.[6]

The illustration shows how officers psychologically move in a circle from whom they were to whom they will eventually become.

Another key to the success of this informal group of officers was realizing that, as a group, each of them had to understand the cause of their pain and that there were recovery processes that could be put in place to help heal the damage done.

Over the years of meeting once a month, the peer support group identified four rules to guide new members when they

Illustration 8.1: The Blue Circle

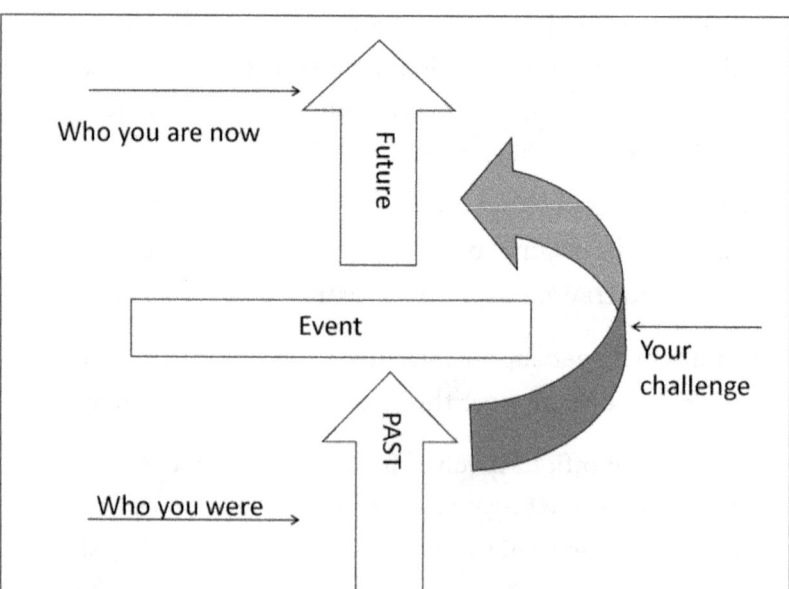

joined. These four rules are quoted here for the benefit of organizations and any potential members who may want to learn what an informal peer team requires from its members.

1. We claim no qualifications other than to have experienced personally the difficulty an officer has in getting reconnected to life after the trauma that we have lived with. .. We deal strictly within the realm of only what we have personally experienced. For members, honesty and trust are crucial.
2. We answer only to the member we are supporting.
3. We advise that, first and foremost, the subject officer should seek professional help at least once to ensure that they are given all the help they need.
4. We assure each member that confidentiality is paramount.[7]

The value of an informal team of peer supporters such as those in the Blue Circle is that its members share a common work-related trauma. They are thus able to empathize with those who seek their support. They listen, provide support and a shoulder to lean on. If they see signs of trauma in a colleague, they are able to direct the officer to the proper professional medical attention. Then they can offer support to them when they admit they need help. Their function is to concentrate on the officer's emotional and mental well-being.

> After starting Robin's Blue Circle, several of the officers assisted in supporting fellow officers often in circumstances that were detrimental to their own careers. Although [this informal peer support was] not accepted initially as a resource by senior [management], members would often be asked by street-level supervisors to respond to calls where officers were involved in shooting incidents. Sometimes, all [they] had to do at first was

show up at work and stand in the hallway, so that a subject officer could see [them] standing there. Just by doing that, the officer knew that they were not alone. As members of the circle, [they] vowed never to leave an officer on their own as they deal with the consequences of a shooting incident.[8]

In today's environment, an informal peer support group can continue to work as has Robin's Blue Circle. But there has to be organizational support for their work. The members of the group must also establish and know their boundaries in offering support. If there is agreement among the members of the group to be empathetic, in positive growth and work hand in hand with professional mental health and trauma-experienced mental health workers, then they should be encouraged by the organization to continue offering support to their colleagues.

No single model of peer support will do everything that is required within an organization. Formal groups, with rules and guidelines, can also include informal groups, which can be set up within the formal structure. Both formal and informal group peers follow the same guidelines and rules, and both can be managed by a formal peer group manager. Although there is much less structure in the informal group setting, they are striving to achieve the same results. The only difference is that informal peers are called on to respond in a way that is entirely outside the boundaries of the organization to meet the needs of a member who does not want support from the formal peer group.

Psychological Testing

Psychological testing and interviewing lived-experience people, who want to become peer supporters, is paramount to ensure that the peer supporter is psychologically ready to help others. This is crucial for a meaningful, safe and ethical program of both informal and formal peer teams.

The purpose of psychological testing is to ensure that the peer does not reactivate their own trauma when helping someone else. It also ensures that the person being helped is not further traumatized by someone who is not ready to provide such help and, thus, should not be in such a trusted relationship with a vulnerable colleague.

There are those who do not believe that peer supporters need to undertake psychological testing. The authors disagree and fully support the need for this testing for anyone with a lived experience of trauma, who wants to become a member of a peer support team. It is essential that peer supporters adhere to the principle of doing no harm to those who seek their support.

Though the authors refer to policing as one of the professions where informal peer groups make the most sense, there is no doubt in their minds that informal peer support groups would work well for any organization.

Peer Support from Brad McKay's Experience

Informal peer support is often an underground and extremely confidential entity that has developed for a reason or a number of reasons. Often these groups develop because the organizations do not have their own program. Or the organization has a program but the employees or members don't trust it.

Peer supporters, whether informal or formal, have no hidden agenda or motives other than to help their own. Informal peer teams develop naturally in a peer-to-peer environment, where there are members from the same discipline who genuinely care enough to support their own confidentially, ethically and through competent skills in a safe and secure environment.

Informal teams should have, where at all possible, trained and experienced leadership, with clinical direction from a competent mental health professional. Opportunities for training and education should be taken when they arise. A high level of trust and credibility is required to provide competent peer support whether it is done informally or through a formal structure. In either case, peer supporters must stay within their boundaries and never do harm intentionally or neglectfully to those seeking their support.

One of the challenges that Brad has seen over the years is that peer supporters can often take on too much emotionally. It is important that they remember and appreciate their empathetic skills and show that they care. As peer supporters, they have the ability to make a significant difference in the life of a colleague and their family. However, their trauma or their mental health challenge is theirs alone. Their journey to wellness cannot take members of the peer team down as well.

Don Kirk and the author started a trauma team at York Regional Police (YRP) in 1989. Don was the sergeant on their tactical team and had been involved in a fatal shooting in 1983. Brad's fatal shooting occurred in 1984. (*See* chapter 13, p. 127.) Both officers were the only ones in the history of YRP to that point who had experienced such a trauma. When some colleagues had similar experiences in the late 1980s, both officers decided to do what they could to support their own.

Don was a confident, seasoned tactical supervisor. Brad was more reserved and still only twenty-five. Neither of them had any training. There were no boundaries or rules, and no formal policies or procedures. Essentially, what they set up was an informal team but it was sanctioned by the police service.

The members they connected with eventually became involved in the evolution of the peer support movement in the York Region. The Trauma Team transitioned into a steering committee in 1995 to form a multiservice CISM team for the region. At first, the York Regional Police did not support this. The York Regional Police Association paid for their training and for creating the manuals. The CISM Team operated essentially as an informal team until 1996, when it evolved into a more formal structure.

This informal team operated through donations and fundraising. It did not get the support of the various emergency services in the area, including the YRP, until it proved itself worthy of their support. Once they saw the value and results of the peer and trauma support, a letter of understanding was drawn up with the service. Then formal procedures and a budget for operation and training were provided.

One thing Brad learned from this experience over those twenty-seven years is that patience, perseverance and a positive attitude—the three P's—are required to achieve a system of peer support that will be used and accepted by all the stakeholders. A functioning formal team cannot be set up overnight. The team needs to build its credibility, while the peer support members continue to do their work. As a result of the persistence, hard work and dedication of all those past team members, a solid formal CISM team has evolved. The team has been registered as a not-for-profit organization, with a complete operating manual to provide direction for its members.

A Caution about Social Media

Many members in first responder services suffering with a mental health challenge or struggling with the symptoms resulting from a trauma exposure are reluctant to turn to their own organization for support because of the ongoing stigma attached to mental illness. Nevertheless, they still want answers. They will often go to the Internet or to social media to search for information and for answers to the issues and trauma they are experiencing. They are also seeking fellowship with like-minded members in similar need.

There are many competent sources of information available. Badge of Life Canada is one such credible organization. However, there are many bogus sites that have been set up by those with no mental health or peer support training; this can be dangerous for an organization's members. The organization needs to caution its employees or members to ask questions when browsing on these sites: Are they operating under written guidelines, policies or procedures? Who are they accountable to? Is there a board of directors? Are they incorporated? A not-for-profit? Do they have liability insurance?

Just because an online organization, or an individual, has hundreds or thousands of followers does not necessarily make them competent or credible. They may appear to be knowledgeable and offer care. Unfortunately, there are crisis junkies and badge, uniform and boot bunnies, as well as hucksters and those with hidden agendas, as well as some with a mental illness of their own which they are working through, who will use any means to regain lost mental health. It is important for both the organization and its peer support teams to provide guidance about these online help sites because there are all kinds of predators online.

Formal Peer Support Teams

When developing a formal peer support team, it is extremely important for an organization to be aware of what its members or employees think. It would be prudent to meet with the leaders of all informal peer support teams under the organization's jurisdiction to get feedback about what the challenges are to developing a more formal system.

Some provinces have a separate agency that investigates and, sometimes, criminally charges police officers where an injury or a death has occurred. As a consequence, police officers may not trust a formal peer support team, if they think that what they say may be subpoenaed and used against them in some way. Lawyers will often advise officers not to tell anyone about the incident in which they were involved, even though working through their trauma experience with a peer and a mental health professional would be extremely helpful to them. This may be one reason why an informal peer support team is more trusted as information is shared in the strictest confidence with colleagues who have been through a similar experience.

There is good news. An organization can develop a formal peer support team that is trusted and it must work hard to maintain that trust. A method of jumpstarting trust is to find candidates who are already seen as reliable and who are trusted by their colleagues. This can be done through the process of peer nomination. (For more information on this staffing process, *see* chapter 9, p. 87.)

CISM versus Peer Support

CISM Teams provide interventions to members who have had a trauma exposure. This is the primary purpose of the CISM model. For organizations wishing to enhance coverage and provide peer support for other mental health challenges, the CISM Team alone will not meet this need. At this point, the organization needs to decide in which direction it wants to go. It can either enhance an existing team with further training, and add peers with a variety of lived experiences, or the organization can create a separate team that will work in partnership with the CISM Team.

Many organizations have a CISM team in place and believe that this is sufficient for all types of peer support. This is not the case, however. While it is true that a CISM team will very likely have the knowledge, skills and ability to provide peer support to the members for a variety of situations, and may already be performing this function now, the team may not meet everyone's need for peer support. The theory behind competent peer support is that a peer supporter should be the best one to understand what a member is going through because of their own lived experience and recovery. Therefore, they can support another member who is struggling with a similar challenge.

In 2014, York Regional Police created a twenty-nine member, in-house Peer Support Team. The York Region CISM Team had been in existence since 1996 and had been providing trauma exposure support to all first responders, that is, police, fire, EMS and hospital emergency department staff. The creation of the in-house YRP team was part of a strategy to enhance efficiency, transition from a reactive to a proactive responder and to support the existing CISM Team. Because the original CISM Team was based on a multidisciplinary system serving more than one organization, YRP needed to create a separate team to ensure proper peer support coverage from within.

The two teams work well together and actually operate from the same office.⁹ An in-house peer support team can provide excellent support to the CISM component. For example, when a serious incident happens to the organization such as the murder or death of one of its members, there will be hours and hours of interventions and group debriefings. The importance of reaching out to each and every member touched by this tragedy is paramount.

One of the more significant findings in the Ontario Ombudsman's report, released in 2012, is that follow-up after any intervention is essential.¹⁰ When dealing with a large-scale event, the organization may not necessarily be aware of how significantly that event has impacted its members. The problem with large-scale events is that it is challenging to provide follow-up when dealing with so many participants.

This is where the Peer Support Team can step in to assist and ensure that each and every participant is contacted. It is important not to let an "us and them" atmosphere develop but to encourage a cooperative working relationship between both sides of the peer support system.

Peer Support Alone

In addition to trauma exposures, there are many areas where peer support can be a major asset to the organization's members. It can provide mental health support to members and their families in times of personal or professional crisis. Through a competent peer support program, the organization can provide its members with the tools to sustain a successful career and a healthy home life. Unmanaged stress can lead to both mental and physical health challenges. It is important to consider all those areas where its members would benefit from peer support. It helps to have as many lived experiences represented on the peer support team as possible. For example, the Peer Support Team may include members who have survived cancer or a serious illness, or who came through a divorce or lost a child. The list of lived experiences is broad and all-encompassing.[11]

Many smaller organizations will find it much easier to blend their CISM and Peer Support Teams so that one unit handles every situation. There is nothing wrong with this, as long as it is understood that the functions and purpose of the teams are different. Peer supporters in a dual role will need to be cross-trained to ensure they have the skills and ability to provide interventions on all fronts where support is required.

Once an organization has determined whether they require a CISM team, an informal or a formal peer support team, the next step will be to determine how these teams should be staffed.

9

Staffing CISM and Peer Support Teams

Whether an organization is staffing a CISM or a peer support team, or a team consisting of both elements, the method is virtually the same. If the organization is fortunate to have a CEO or chief who supports mental health wellness strategies, reducing the stigma of mental illness, and creating quality peer support, then the organization has a major head start in staffing these peer teams.

There can be barriers when CISM or peer support is labeled as the chief's initiative, or team, and the front line ranks will not likely trust teams labeled as such. Nor will there be much trust from the front lines if these teams are created by a human resources department or set up by the union or member association.[1]

Getting Started

The road to success in staffing a CISM and peer support team rests with whomever is creating the team and staffing it. There must be a peer support leader, someone on the front lines who is trusted by them. This person needs to be transparent, ethical and dedicated to the well-being of both the organization and the members. This person needs to be trusted by the CEO and by the heads of the union or association. This person will be the one to drive any strategy to create the team and then to staff it.

DETERMINING THE LEADER

The Mental Health Commission of Canada has recommended that an individual with a lived experience, who is in a healthy state of recovery, is best suited to be a peer supporter in their organization. A lived experience survivor will likely be most suited for the lead role. This person must be willing to share his or her journey to show others they are not alone and that the new program will reduce the stigma associated with mental illness and provide resources for wellness. This person should have the flexibility to perform this volunteer function as leader, in addition to the regular assigned duties. But the time will come when the organization needs to step up and cover the time spent providing support and setting up the system. And the CEO will need to make this happen.

CREATING A WORKING GROUP OR COMMITTEE

The leader, along with a number of stakeholders who are invested and passionate about creating a healthy work environment within the organization, should form the Steering Committee or Working Group. Committee work can be long, exhaustive and unproductive at times. It is necessary to find representatives from various areas in the organization including a senior officer or manager, the union or association president, a nurse or other lead person in the health and wellness section of human resources, a community mental health liaison member, a psychologist or mental health professional from the organization or community, and a middle manager or supervisor in a high-risk unit (e.g., Internet child exposure) in the organization.

THE SUBJECT MATTER EXPERT (SME)

A subject matter expert (SME) is someone who has significant knowledge and experience, and has created a peer-driven team in their organization with a significant degree of success. There are organizations that have created very successful peer support systems. As an example, the Mood Disorders Society of Canada, based in Ottawa, has a peer and trauma support systems group with SMEs that can help the steering committee.

The committee members need to ask the SME for a step-by-step explanation of how their team was created, what worked and what didn't. The committee should also ask what could have been done differently. The process to be followed should meet the organization's unique needs to create a successful CISM and peer support team. After learning as much as possible from the SME, it is important to stay connected in case there are more questions.

ANNOUNCING THE INITIATIVE TO THE ORGANIZATION

Because setting up a peer support system is a significant step, which the organization is taking, the Steering Committee should announce this initiative and make this a reason for the members or employees to celebrate. (*See* chapter 3 for more information on how to create a communications strategy; the steps are essentially the same.) Any announcement that is to be made should come from the leader. At this same time, the message to be communicated should ensure everyone that the Peer and/or CISM Team is an initiative being driven from the frontline ranks.

If the organization has intranet or a web-based network, information can be shared on it by posting notices about the committee, its work and the goal to be achieved. This also provides an opportunity to seek feedback from the stakeholders who may have experience in trauma recovery. Information sessions can be held during pre-shift briefings.

The Steering Committee needs to review the feedback provided by employees and contact those who sent their ideas or suggestions. Whether their ideas are viable or not, it is still important for the committee to look at their concerns and review their ideas. After all, the CISM/Peer Support Program is being set up for the members; their opinions must count and their concerns heard.

The committee should then ask for the program champion—the chief or CEO—to make a statement of support and appreciation for the program. This assures the workforce that the program will be driven and operated by the front line and its integrity and confidentiality respected. This message can be in the weekly or monthly organizational publication. This same message of support should also come from the head of the union or member association.

Ongoing communication from the leader of the Steering Committee is important throughout the staffing process or for however long the committee exists to keep the front lines informed about what progress is being made, the next steps to be taken, the timelines for the staffing process and what the anticipated size of the Peer Support Team will be. Keeping the workforce informed about all the steps the committee has taken to get buy-in from the members is important and ensures the organization that the committee is being as transparent as possible about what it is doing.

Staffing the Team

It is best to have representation from as many areas of the organization as possible on the CISM and Peer Support Team. Staffing a team involves four steps.

STEP 1 – THE NOMINATION PROCESS

One of the pioneers in the peer nomination method is the Tema Conter Memorial Trust, based in King City, Ontario. Its current director is Vince Savoia and, along with co-author McKay, they sat on an interview panel for two greater Toronto area (GTA) frontline emergency service organizations to select their peer team members. Each of the candidates had been nominated for the position by their peers. The same selection method was used as that for the in-house Peer Support Team at York Regional Police.

Candidates are nominated because someone they work with believes in their ability to support others. The candidates have likely shown that they have compassion, ability and the credibility required to provide support. And more than likely they are already providing support. All they may lack is the training, experience and clinical direction.

Candidates, who are serious about peer support and who are already providing it in an informal setting, may already have taken some training on their own. They are ideal candidates for a formal peer support team. Peer nomination is the best way to identify and harness them for the team. Knowing that the organization supports the peer support team both financially and by setting up a formal structure, without breaching guaranteed confidentiality, gives members confidence that their organization cares about their well-being.

Posting the Notice: When posting for candidates, the notice should be both clear and precise as to what the committee is seeking in candidates. The Notice of Peer Support Opportunity should indicate how many positions will be filled, that peers will be chosen based on their lived experience, their position in the organization, where they work and where they live. The posting should also indicate who they will report to. It is important to let potential candidates know that the committee is seeking a cross-section of nominees. The notice should be posted for at least two weeks to ensure that all potential nominators have the opportunity to see it.

Qualifications: The posting should also include what qualifications are required for a peer support member. These qualifications include good interpersonal communication skills in order to build honest, nonjudgmental and trusting peer relationships. Critical thinking skills will assist the peer in understanding the issues being discussed. The ability to work in a team environment, especially for CISM peers, is important as some interventions occur in a group setting. A person who has shown integrity and is known to be ethical will bring this to the peer relationship. Perhaps, the most important qualification is that the nominee has a lived experience of a mental health challenge, which they have survived and are now in the positive stages of growth and health.

Requirements of the Position: The position will require that candidates be nominated by someone in the organization. The candidates must agree to attend training (the initial training dates should be listed), pass the course and attend meetings when required. They must be highly motivated, with good time management skills in order to handle peer support duties as well as their regular assigned duties. The candidate must have at least three years' experience with the organization. They must agree to and participate in a psychological test and an interview with a psychologist. The candidate must be someone in good standing with the organization and who is capable of maintaining confidentiality about the nature of the peer support provided.

The Nominator's Responsibility: The nominator should complete a short questionnaire that includes their name, the name of the nominee and nominee's number of years of service. The nominator must indicate how long they have known the nominee, whether they discussed the nomination with the nominee and if the nominee is interested in being a peer. The nominator should be asked to describe why they believe the nominee would be a good candidate, if this person is trusted within the organization and why. Finally, the nominator must give an example of when they have seen the nominee providing peer support to someone.

Acknowledging the Nominations: As nominations are received, the leader should review them. The next steps include: 1) contacting the candidate to confirm that they are interested in participating in the interview and selection process; 2) ensuring the candidate can attend the mandatory training; and 3) has been employed with the organization for at least three years; 4) determining their home address and, finally; 5) asking the organization if there are any behaviour or disciplinary concerns.

STEP 2 – PSYCHOLOGICAL TESTING AND ASSESSMENT

The next step in the selection process is to ask all candidates to undergo psychological testing and assessment. (This is known as safeguarding. *See* chapter 6, p. 54.) If for some reason, it is determined that a candidate is not psychologically healthy at this time to be a peer supporter, this can be decided collaboratively with the candidate and the mental health professional. This decision is made in confidence and only known by them. The benefit of doing the testing at this stage is that the candidate can withdraw from the process without any explanation or questions asked.

The psychologist should be experienced and comfortable in administering and reviewing the results of these tests. They should already be experienced in providing therapy to members in the organization. They should also have a good understanding of the roles and responsibilities of the organization's members and the jargon used in the work environment.

The psychologist will have a routine set of questions for the candidate including demographics and background, family and candidate medical and psychiatric history, medications, exercise routines, sleep, and stress strategies, among others. The psychologist will focus on any red flags that surface in the testing that was administered. What the psychologist also needs to do is take this opportunity to prepare the candidate mentally for the task of being a peer supporter.

In some larger organizations, the recruitment unit will have accounts with psychological testing providers with the ability to administer the testing online and to provide proper instruction to the candidates. If this is the case, it will save time and money; the candidates can take the test ahead of time, so that they can attend the interview with the psychologist a few days later. This gives the psychologist time to review the test before meeting with the candidate. If the organization doesn't have online access to testing, then a psychologist will need to set it up for the candidate; this may be a written test that will have to be reviewed before an assessment can be made.

Any areas of concern that surface as a result of testing will need to be addressed with the candidate by the mental health professional. They will not be discussed with the lead. This provides confidentiality and protection for the candidate and lends credibility to the program. The psychologist alone will determine if the candidate is psychologically healthy and suitable to be a peer supporter. If the psychologist determines that the candidate is not suitable at that time, this will be conveyed to the candidate and the candidate will agree to withdraw from the process. On a rare occasion, a candidate may refuse to withdraw. This is the only circumstance under which the psychologist will brief the lead to ensure the candidate is removed from the process and, at the same time, ensure that there is support for this person, if needed.

There are a number of psychological tests available from a variety of providers.[2] The organization may have a psychologist on staff or on contract who is familiar with the various tests.

Some organizations will rely solely on the psychologist to make a decision without administering any tests. While this can be a cost-saving for the organization, it reduces the number of tools available to assist in making the best assessment and puts significant responsibility on the psychologist. It is recommended that the organization either purchase psychological tests from a provider or ask the psychologist about testing; the mental health provider may already have an account with a company that provides these tests.

There have been discussions about the need psychologically to assess members who will be performing peer support duties. The Mental Health Commission of Canada has indicated that, "The primary personal attribute necessary to provide quality peer support is lived experience with a mental health challenge or illness (either personally or through a loved one), accompanied by the experience of finding a path of recovery."[3]

Peer team candidates will likely have had a lived experience with a mental health challenge. Members of the selection committee should always keep in mind that enhancing the well-being of members should never be achieved at the cost of the peer supporters. There are risks in not conducting psychological testing. However, it is the view of both authors that peer support is a higher-risk position that could challenge the mental health of a peer supporter. Therefore, it is of the utmost importance to ensure that all candidates are mentally healthy before taking on a peer support role.

STEP 3 – THE INTERVIEW

In conducting the interview, it may be appropriate to invite an outside peer supporter to sit on the interview team or panel.[4] The benefit of having an outsider on the panel is that they are experienced and knowledgeable; however, they are not connected to the organization and can be more objective. They are unaware of inside rumours and gossip about specific individuals and will conduct an unbiased interview. A good interviewer from an outside agency can praise the candidate for their commitment to the wellness of their own members, as well as the organization for setting up a peer program.

The ideal interview panel will consist of two to three interviewers with at least one from an outside organization.

The other interviewer is the leader or a trusted designate from within the organization. The interview should not exceed thirty minutes. The following questions are suggested, each of which can be rated on a scale of one to five:

1. What is your understanding of peer support and why do you want to be a part of the team?
2. What would you do if you learned a coworker was making suicidal comments?
3. When have you provided peer support? (Provide an example.)
4. What attributes would your friends describe in you that would benefit a peer support team?
5. What training and education do you have that would benefit your role in peer support?
6. How would you rate yourself in terms of conduct and credibility?

At the conclusion of the interview, the interviewers can come to an agreement on the scoring. Or they can do their own scoring and average it. The scoring will be helpful for the next step.

STEP 4 — SELECTING QUALIFIED PEER SUPPORTERS

Once the interviews are completed, it is time to look at all the candidates from a number of perspectives. If selecting someone for a peer support team and not specifically for a CISM team, then one other important category needs to be determined and that is the type of lived experience of each candidate. The following categories will also determine the most successful candidates for the peer support team.

Interview Score: A high interview score will mean that this candidate is likely already performing informal peer support. Therefore, those with high scores should be given more consideration. A person with a lower score is not necessarily ineligible for the team; it simply means that the high-score candidate already has much of the mindset of a quality team member.

Location of Regular Duties: Some organizations have more than one office, building or district and are spread out across municipalities, provinces or the country. When selecting candidates for a team, it is important to have peer support representation at each location if possible. This makes it easier to respond to needs in the workplace in a timely manner.

Type of Duties: It is especially important to have peer support members who have worked, or are working, in some of the higher-risk areas of the organization, if possible. Their work experience in areas at a higher risk of exposure to trauma or death will enhance the peer team.

Area of Residence: Often peer support is provided after work hours so there may be a need to meet a member at or near their residence. In many organizations, especially in Canadian urban centres, members may have to commute considerable distance. It is important to keep this in mind when selecting peers. Having a cross-section of peers who live in the areas where many of the organization's employees work will be helpful in deploying peer support and when connecting the member and family to professional resources.

Type of Lived Experience: It is imperative that, in the early stages of developing a peer support team, there is a variety of trauma exposure experience and other significant experiences. Peer supporters who have specific experience will likely have credibility in the area of their own lived experience. Peer members can have experience with shootings, the death or murder of children or a coworker, mass casualties, suicide and so on. As peer team members build trust, get training and gain experience, their credibility will grow and they will be able to help many others who need support in the organization.

Additional Peer Support Members

Although the best members for a peer support team can be found within the organization, this doesn't mean that the focus should only be on the organization's members with peer support experience. There are others with different life experiences who may also enhance the peer support or CISM team.

COMMUNICATORS

Those who staff a call centre/radio room in a first responder organization are, in many cases, the true first responder. These frontline communicators will actually hear threats, panic and fear, and possibly violent acts occurring that result in death. Communicators are the link to ensure that information about the incident is being effectively sent to the responders. Communicators experience high levels of stress, anxiety and the effects of trauma from not knowing what is happening at the site of the call.

To say that communicators are required on a peer support team or a CISM team is an understatement. They are an essential part of the first responder organization and are often forgotten. They need to be valued for their necessary contribution and, where possible, included in any intervention as part of the CISM Team.

Bruce Herridge, current director of the Ontario Police College, managed the Communications Branch as an inspector at York Regional Police.[5] After training, he became a member of the York Region CISM Team. He advocated for the members in his branch to ensure that they were cared for and supported at the same level as frontline responders. Soon, more communicators were added to the team and interventions were being provided to communications people.

CHAPLAINS

Spiritual leaders in communities are highly respected. Their training, education and experience enable them to deal with their congregation who are in personal, professional or family crisis. As specialists in dealing with death and bereavement, they can be a natural addition to an organization's peer support system.

Often they are underutilized and restricted to attending special functions, photo opportunities or delivering the blessing. For chaplains to be effective, they need to have a significant understanding of the organization, the work environment and the workforce. Ride-a-longs and visits are beneficial so that the members can get to know them.

The chaplain, or the rabbi, priest, imam or minister, is viewed as a trusted confidential avenue to share challenges and mitigate stress. There is little stigma associated with sitting down and having a chat with them. This means the chaplain can be a huge asset in many ways. They can assist when a serious event occurs such as the sudden death of a member. The chaplain can provide a unique perspective when accompanying a mental health professional or peer supporter, or when doing an intervention. They are comfortable entering the family home to provide assistance. They can meet and address a group of members who are at a loss as to why a tragedy occurred. They can encourage respectful dialogue and can inject a spiritual perspective when asked or required to do so.

FAMILY

It is important to have family representation on the Peer Support Team. Spousal peer supporters and significant others provide significant benefits to peer support systems. The family, more often than not, is the first to notice a change in a member who is suffering from a mental health challenge.

Spouses of first responders often work in the same organization. They know the organization and the family dynamics in supporting a spouse with a lived experience of a mental health challenge. They may have survived their own lived experience and are in a position of positive growth. Family member candidates may already be advocating and supporting others. A selection committee should consider adding them to the Peer Support Team. (There is an excellent model of family support known as Beyond the Blue.)[6]

SENIOR OFFICERS

Bruce Herridge was the first senior officer to be trained in CISM. He was on a peer support team as a peer to York Regional Police senior officers in need. This is a complicated situation, as members consider having a senior manager on a peer support team as jeopardizing the team's credibility.

As a senior officer, Bruce Herridge maintained a low profile and only attended meetings and training when urgently required. He also assisted with fundraising and stepped up as the master of ceremonies at significant events. He always respected the high level of confidentiality required for interventions by the CISM Team. He is the model of how a senior officer can be a significant asset to a peer support system, while working quietly behind the scene.

RETIRED MEMBERS

The Peer Support Team may want to consider adding retired members of the organization to the team. Having a junior retired member available for this group shows that the members care about them in retirement. Retired members on the peer support team add a level of trust because they are no longer accountable to the organization. Retired members, who dedicate their time to peer support, will more likely be trusted by senior officers or managers and are seen as serving the needs of the member only.

This chapter has provided information that makes it easier for an organization to select peer team members.

10

Organizational Training for CISM and Peer Support Teams

Every organization of frontline responders and service providers has potential peer supporters within it. And, when it comes to helping the organization's staff or members, who may be in crisis or suffering silently from an unacknowledged trauma, there is no one better suited than a trusted peer, that is, a colleague who sincerely cares and who has experienced a similar event or trauma. Whether peer supporters are operating in a formal, structured system that includes a CISM team, or in an informal group, it is imperative that essential training and education be provided.

Formal peer supporters and members of CISM teams need to know what they are doing so that their members don't unintentionally do more harm than good. If the organization or first responder service has established a formal peer support/CISM system for its workforce, then it must ensure that the individuals who are peer supporters are competent, capable, ethical and clinically supervised. Most importantly, they should be trained and certified.

Organizational Training Resources

It can be very confusing for an organization to determine what training is suitable for peer supporters in order to give them the tools they need to provide the best possible support for their colleagues when it is needed.

Some believe that a Critical Incident Stress Management (CISM) team, with training provided by the International Critical Incident Stress Foundation, is sufficient to provide peer support. Others believe that general peer support training is sufficient for trauma intervention, when a person within the service has been exposed to a traumatic event.

This is not the case, however. There must be a clear distinction between peer support required after a trauma exposure and general peer support for staff or members, who are experiencing a mental health challenge for reasons not necessarily related to a work trauma exposure. It is possible that a mental health challenge can surface, which could eventually be attributed to a trauma exposure or to PTSD. Wherever possible, it is always better for the service to have peer supporters in place who can provide assistance to those who are dealing with a similar lived experience, with the necessary training.

There are many resources, workshops and courses available from recognized organizations to train and certify peer supporters in a number of fields. The authors have provided a quick reference table (*see* table 10.1). It lists the various organizations that provide information on creating a workplace environment that is mentally healthy. The quick reference table also includes the organizations and the training and certification, as well as ongoing education that they provide to members of peer support and CISM teams.

Table 10.1: A Quick Reference Sheet

A Quick Reference Sheet developed for the support of peer and trauma systems by the Mood Disorders Society of Canada Peer Support Services Team	Guarding Minds @ Work	R2MR for Police and Military	Anti-Stigma Campaigns	Peer Support Services, Mood Disorders Society of Canada	Living Works Canada or Canadian Critical Incident Stress Foundation	Tema Conter	National Organization for Victims Assistance	Association of Traumatic Stress Specialists
Determining Current Status								
Current 13 Psychosocial Strengths /Gaps	√							
Introductory Awareness and Resiliency workshops								
Resiliency and Trauma Awareness Training (members and leaders)		√		√				
Resiliency and Trauma Awareness Training (families)		√		√				
Suicide Awareness (members and leaders)					√			
Suicide Awareness (families)					√			
Anti-Stigma Campaign								
Anti-Stigma Campaign			√					
Essential Training and Certification for Peer Support Groups								
Peer Support Training Workshop				√				
Suicide Prevention, Intervention, and Postvention Training Workshop					√			
Individual Crisis and Peer Support Workshop					√			
Group Crisis Intervention					√			
Mental Health First Aid						√		
Advanced Group Crisis Intervention					√			
Crisis Response Training							√	
Advanced Crisis Response Training							√	
Ongoing Education and Certifications								
Certified Trauma Responder								√
Certified Trauma Specialist								√
Certified Trauma Services Specialist								√
Ongoing Updates on Research, Journals, Articles and Findings.	Develop a common link between all active mental wellness members to share information							

Recommended training can be categorized into four areas as follows:
1. Essential Training for All Members of Peer Support Teams, Including CISM Teams
2. Essential Training Specific to Members of CISM Teams
3. Recommended Training for All Members of Peer Support Teams, Including CISM Teams
4. Recommended Certification for Members of Peer Support and CISM Teams to Validate Training and Competency

1. ESSENTIAL TRAINING FOR ALL MEMBERS OF PEER SUPPORT TEAMS, INCLUDING CISM TEAMS

A. Peer and Trauma Support System (PATSS): Two-day Peer Support Training, Accredited by the Mood Disorders Society of Canada

In 2013, the Mental Health Commission of Canada (MHCC) published *Guidelines for the Practice and Training of Peer Support*.[1] These guidelines were used by the Mood Disorders Society of Canada to develop P.A.T.S.S. This is an evidenced-based, seventeen-module, two-day training curriculum that matches the exact objectives as provided in the MHCC's guidelines.

The two-day, accredited training course is formatted directly from the guidelines and addresses the following three themes:
1. Fundamental Principals of Peer Support
2. Social and Historical Context of Peer Support
3. Concepts and Methods That Promote Peer-to-Peer Effectiveness

The modules cover seventeen subjects and consist of the following:

Module 1.1 Lived Experience, Hope, and Recovery

Module 1.2 Self-Determination and How to Foster It
Module 1.3 Peer Support Values, Ethics and Principles of Practice
Module 1.4 Trauma-Informed Practice
Module 1.5 Applying Peer Support Principles in Diverse Environments
Module 2.1 The Historical Context of Peer Support
Module 2.2 Prejudice, Discrimination and Stigma
Module 2.3 Diversity and Social Inclusion
Module 2.4 Social Determinants of Health
Module 3.1 Interpersonal Communication Principles and Methods
Module 3.2 Building Supportive Relationships
Module 3.3 The Process of Recovery and Change
Module 3.4 Building Resilience Through Self-Care and Wellness Plans
Module 3.5 Limits and Boundaries
Module 3.6 Crisis Situations and Strategies
Module 3.7 Connecting with Community Resources
Module 3.8 Awareness of Possible Symptoms and Potential Side Effects of Medication

B. LivingWorks Education: Applied Suicide Intervention Skills Training (ASIST): Two-day Suicide Intervention Training Workshop

LivingWorks Education is the world leader in providing training for suicide intervention. ASIST "is the world's leading suicide intervention workshop."[2] Developed in 1983 by LivingWorks, a company based in Australia, with branches in Canada and the United States, ASIST teaches

> suicide first aid. Shown by major studies to significantly reduce suicidality, the ASIST model teaches effective intervention skills while helping to build suicide prevention networks in the community.

Suicide intervention skills are essential learning for all peer support workers in order to identify the risk factors and know how to engage and be comfortable with that uncomfortable and essential conversation.[3]

2. ESSENTIAL TRAINING SPECIFIC TO MEMBERS OF CISM TEAMS

A. International Critical Incident Stress Foundation, Inc. (ICISF): Assisting Individuals in Crisis: Two-day Course

The ICISF is an American organization that provides "leadership, education, training, consultation and support services in . . . crisis intervention. . . ."[4] (The equivalent in Canada is the Canadian Critical Incident Stress Foundation located in Hamilton.) It offers a number of certificate specialized training programs. The Assisting Individuals in Crisis certificate program is described as follows:

> Crisis intervention is NOT psychotherapy; rather, it is a specialized acute emergency mental health intervention which requires special training. As physical first aid is to surgery, crisis intervention is to psychotherapy. Thus, crisis intervention is sometimes called "emotional first aid". This program is designed . . . for anyone who desires to increase their knowledge of individual (one-on-one) crisis intervention techniques in the fields of Business & Industry, Crisis Intervention, Disaster Response, Education, Emergency Services, Employee Assistance, Healthcare, Homeland Security, Mental Health, Military, Spiritual Care, and Traumatic Stress.[5]

B. International Critical Incident Stress Foundation, Inc. (ICISF): Group Crisis Intervention: Two- day Course

> Designed to present the core elements of a comprehensive, systematic and multi-component crisis intervention curriculum, the Group Crisis Intervention course will prepare

participants to understand a wide range of crisis intervention services. Fundamentals of Critical Incident Stress Management (CISM) will be outlined and participants will leave with the knowledge and tools to provide several group crisis interventions, specifically demobilizations, defusings, and the Critical Incident Stress Debriefing (CISD). The need for appropriate follow-up services and referrals when necessary will also be discussed.

This course is designed for anyone in the fields of Business & Industry Crisis Intervention, Disaster Response, Education, Emergency Services, Employee Assistance, Healthcare, Homeland Security, Mental Health, Military, Spiritual Care, and Traumatic Stress.[6]

These two courses are also available in a three-day combination training package.

3. RECOMMENDED TRAINING FOR ALL MEMBERS OF PEER SUPPORT TEAMS, INCLUDING CISM TEAMS

A. The Tema Conter Memorial Trust: MANERS Psychological First Aid Training: Two-day Workshop

Developed by Victorian Ambulance Services in Australia, MANERS has been adapted from a psychological first aid model called SAFER; this, in turn, was developed by George Everly out of the Mitchell debriefing model. "The aim of Psychological First Aid is to provide early and supportive interventions, which will assist people with the emotional distress that may result from their involvement in an accident, injury, or sudden shocking event."[7]

MANERS is a crisis intervention model that may be used when dealing with individuals involved in a critical or traumatic event. MANERS is the acronym for a model of psychological first aid that incorporates the following six stages:

> M – Minimize exposure
>
> A – Acknowledge the response and/or event
>
> N – Normalize the response or reaction
>
> E – Educate as required
>
> R – Restore or Refer
>
> S – Self care

B. International Critical Incident Stress Foundation: Advanced Group Crisis Intervention Course

Designed to provide participants with the latest information on critical incident stress management techniques and post-trauma syndromes, the Advanced Group Crisis Intervention builds on the knowledge base which was obtained through the Group Crisis Intervention course and/or in publications. At the conclusion of the course, participants will have been exposed to specific, proven strategies to intervene with those suffering the ill effects of their exposure to trauma. Emphasis will be on advanced defusings and debriefings in complex situations. This course is designed for EAP, human resources and public safety personnel, mental health professionals, chaplains, emergency medical services providers, firefighters, physicians, police officers, nurses, dispatchers, airline personnel and disaster workers who are already trained in the critical incident stress debriefing format. It will also be useful for those working extensively with traumatized victims for various walks of life. This course requires previous training and experience. ICISF's "Group Crisis Intervention" should be viewed as a prerequisite.[8]

B. International Critical Incident Stress Foundation: Suicide Prevention, Intervention, and Postvention Course

Why do people kill themselves? How do I ask someone if they are feeling suicidal? What do I do if they say they ARE suicidal? How do I deal with the strong emotions suicide generates? This course will provide answers for these and other questions many . . . crisis interventionists have about suicide. It will provide participants with basic information about suicide as well as help participants develop practical skills for prevention, intervention and postvention. Small group role plays will allow participants to apply the suggested techniques as they are learned.

This course is open to anyone who wishes to learn more about intervening across the suicide spectrum. Professionals from the fields of Business & Industry Crisis Intervention, Disaster Response, Education, Emergency Services, Employee Assistance, Healthcare, Homeland Security, Mental Health, Military, Spiritual Care, and Traumatic Stress may all benefit.[9]

C. National Organization for Victim Assistance (NOVA): Community Crisis Response Team Training

The purpose of NOVA crisis response and intervention curriculum is to assist individuals, groups and communities to develop, utilize and build on their natural resources of strength and resilience in the emotional aftermath of a disaster. This curriculum and its accompanying training seek to address the theory, skills and team development needed for establishing and maintaining an effective Community Crisis Response Team.[10]

4. RECOMMENDED CERTIFICATION FOR MEMBERS OF PEER SUPPORT AND CISM TEAMS TO VALIDATE TRAINING AND COMPETENCY

A. Association of Traumatic Stress Specialists (ATSS): Certified Trauma Responder, Certified Trauma Services Specialist, Certified Trauma Treatment Specialist

The ATSS, located in South Carolina, is membership-based. It provides its members with the opportunity to become recognized for their certification in a trauma specialty.[11] In order to be certified by ATSS, individuals must be members of the association.

> The **Certified Trauma Responder (CTR)** designation was created for first responders and others who provide immediate trauma intervention through individual and group crisis intervention, critical incident stress response, debriefing, crisis and disaster management, peer counseling, disaster and trauma response, and follow up.
>
> The **Certified Trauma Services Specialist (CTSS)** - created for individuals who provide services and support to individuals impacted by traumatic events; who provide immediate trauma intervention, advocacy, crisis intervention, death notification, victim/survivor assistance and immediate and longer-term services for a variety of traumatized populations. This designation also recognizes treatment specialists who focus on multiple services to victims, in addition to treatment and specialized interventions.
>
> The **Certified Trauma Treatment Specialist (CTTS),** a designation for counselors, clinicians, and treatment specialists who provide immediate and longer-term individual, group, and/or family counseling, therapy, grief counseling or support to trauma survivors either as a specialty or within their field of practice.[12]

Organizational Training

Organizations, and especially first responder services, need to invest in offering the necessary training and certification for members of Peer Support and CISM Teams. This will give a measure of confidence to employees, or members, that those who are providing support and intervention are qualified to do so.

11

How a CISM and Peer Support System Can Work

Since each organization is unique in terms of its need for a peer support system, there is no single template that provides all the strategies and tools needed to give direction on how a peer support or CISM system will work. It is best to speak to several organizations within the same discipline to view their policies and procedures. First responder services have different requirements to operate effectively for their organization.[1]

Where there is an established peer support and/or CISM team, there will likely be people within the organization willing to share their methods and strategies, and operational manuals. The organization should review as many documents as possible from similar organizations or services.

Selecting Strategies and Tools

There are many ways in which first responder services and organizations can assist their peer support and CISM teams to be effective partners in the work environment to ensure that the workforce is mentally healthy. Many of these accommodate the philosophy to be proactive, rather than reactive, and to ensure no harm comes to those who are employed by the organization. This is not possible for every organization as some services or agencies—due to the nature of their mandate—are in the business of sending their members into harm's way. But, if they have already set up their peer support and CISM teams, then there are many strategies that the organization can invest in to assist their peer support system in being even more effective. A first step is to become proactive.

REACTIVE TO PROACTIVE STRATEGIES

What leading-edge organizations are now doing is transitioning from a reactive model of peer support to a proactive one. They are learning that the earlier mental health challenges and work-related traumas are identified and addressed in the workplace, the shorter the road to wellness will be. Employers know "that there is a human cost when employees with mental health illnesses don't get help.... Employers also know that unaddressed mental illness affects productivity and costs companies' money."[2]

Early intervention is the key. There are a number of strategies that can assist an organization in detecting potential mental health challenges in the workforce. All of these can be driven either by the peer support team or the wellness department. Early intervention provides the first responder service with the opportunity to interact with a member or employee in need before a serious behaviour or disciplinary problem occurs. With the member's permission, the organization can offer support to the family. Through peer support, mental health resources and a team effort, the member can be assisted in the journey to recovery and regaining mental health.

EARLY INTERVENTION STRATEGIES

Implementing early intervention strategies can be an effective way for the organization to become proactive in dealing with workplace mental health challenges and trauma. But it is essential that there is an easy way for employees to contact someone when they do seek help. The more complex the system, the less likely a member will use it.

Ease of Contact: Usually, the first point of contact starts with a phone call. When a member has the courage to call for help, it can be the most frightening step they have taken. The organization needs to create a reliable first point of contact where each person is treated with compassion, care and respect.

Illustration 11.1: Supportive Hands

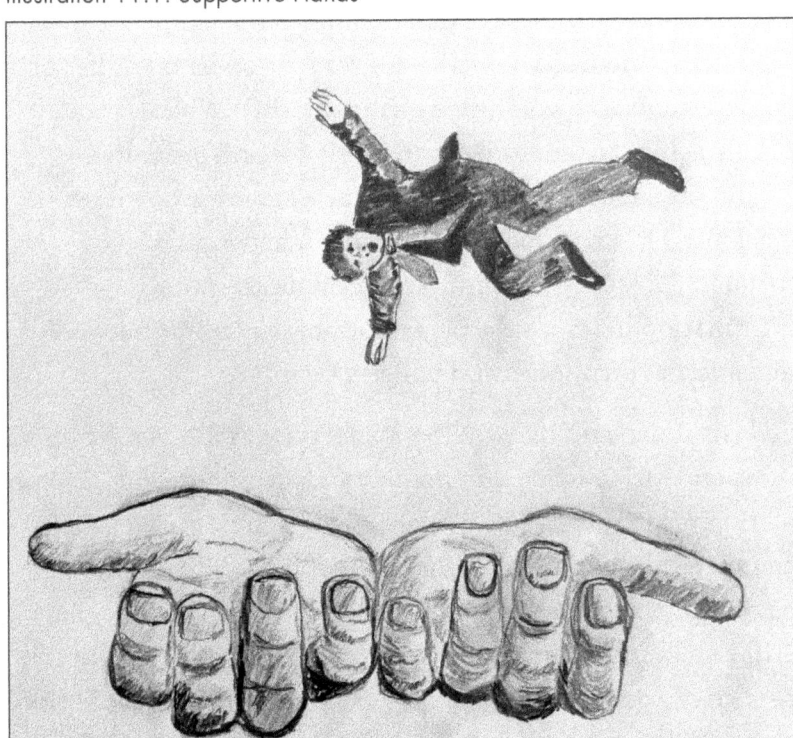

This sketch shows how peer support works by being there to catch a falling member.

They need to know that they can trust this person and that their conversation is confidential. In fact, the person designated as the first point of contact must be consistent, fair and effective to anyone who reaches out.

When adopting this strategy, the organization needs to be aware of the fact that this responsibility is exhausting and too much for one individual to handle on their own. These calls may occur at all hours of the day and night, and during vacation time. This responsibility of first contact needs to be shared among senior members and leaders of the peer support team. The coordinator of the team will need to schedule each member of the team as a designated contact.

Sometimes teams will use a central email or voicemail service. The problem with these contact points is that someone may be in crisis and need immediate intervention, and neither of these systems can guarantee confidentiality. Whatever point of contact is chosen, it needs to be visible and promoted within the organization so that employees are aware if its existence. Promotional tools may include pens, fridge magnets, posters in lunchrooms or on lockers, the information index on the organization's electronic network, and stickers on phones and bulletin boards.

Toll Free Number: The York Regional Police (YRP) has set up an independent, toll-free number, not only for police but also for all first responder services under its jurisdiction. To ensure complete confidentiality, YRP contracted with the same service provider that monitors the calls for the York Region crime stoppers program. The benefit of using this type of service provider enables the organization to provide specifics about what is needed. For example, the specifics can include: eliminate or keep call identifier; take information and forward as a group text or email to the intervention coordinators so that an immediate call-back can be made; include specific individuals such as the clinical director; or patch through to the cell phone of the team member on call. This is an excellent method of trusted contact. It is cost-effective and the service can be shared with other jurisdictions to save money.

Family Partners: Family members will be an important part of the partnership in the peer support system. The organization needs to consider including them in the wellness strategy. They are the first people to see changes in the behaviour of the organization's employees. (It has already been suggested that family members be included on any peer support team. *See* chapter 9, p. 97).

Illustration 11.2: Reaching Out

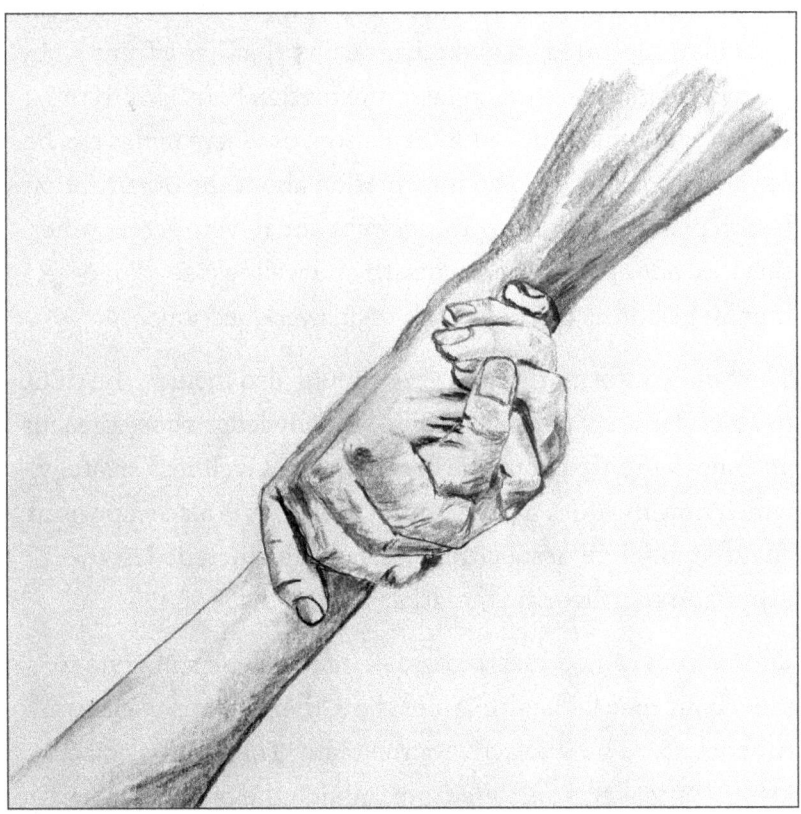

This sketch shows someone reaching out and finding support.

The family needs to know how to reach out for peer support not only for their loved one but also for themselves. Information on how to contact the team can be sent home in pay envelopes. It can be listed in organizational or association/union publications that are likely shared with the family. Early intervention means there will be a better chance of not only helping a member but also saving a marriage and protecting children, who can be very vulnerable when the home environment becomes toxic.

Early intervention methods should also include providing valuable knowledge to the family itself. Appropriate promotional tools can be used to inform the family about the annual family information evening. Family members of high school age and over can be invited to a two-hour session. It can be held in a lecture hall or similar facility that has a front lobby or foyer that can accommodate information booths with the EAP provider handing out information, or where tables can be set up with brochures and information about the organization's health plan, its psychological services and how to access other services. Someone from the health and wellness section or human resources can be on-site to answer questions.

The family information evening should also include the CEO, or chief. He can open the session, acknowledge those present and speak briefly about the organization's wellness strategy, which now includes a peer support team. It is also important that the union or association president be included in the event and in delivering remarks.

Others who can be asked to speak may include someone to talk about mental health issues, how the peer support team functions and how to activate the team. There can also be a keynote speaker, someone from outside the organization who can speak from their own lived experience. A spouse of a member who lost their life on duty is a good choice or an adult child who lost a parent. A fitness specialist or dietician can make a short presentation on the importance of physical health to overall wellness. Motivational videos can be shown just prior to the closing remarks.

EARLY INTERVENTION ANALYST

Establishing the position of an early intervention analyst can be the most significant asset an organization invests in to transition from a reactive to a proactive peer support system. This analyst may have a similar skill set to that of a crime analyst. Having an early intervention analyst with lived experience is even more beneficial to the organization. Because of their lived experience, this analyst will likely be highly dedicated and driven to identify the risk factors needed to help the Peer Support Team make the appropriate decision about how to connect to an employee who may be in need.

Analysts usually have access to tools and data to conduct searches for specific information that the organization and its peer support team will need to identify those employees most at risk of a work-related trauma or a mental health injury. Usually, the organization has a record management system. With the assistance of technicians and programmers, the analyst can define the boundaries for collecting specific information that will be useful in proactively identifying members in need. Information such as the top ten call-outs for first responder services can be invaluable in identifying risk factors for members.[3]

With this type of information, the Peer Support or CISM Team will be aware of the need for an intervention or for a peer supporter to engage with the member. Weekly reports can be automatically generated by the records management system to ensure that information is provided to the analyst and lead peer, so that a more thorough review of the report can be completed. Hospitals may be interested in how many deaths their staff are exposed to. Financial institutions such as banks may want to know how many assaultive or aggressive customers their customer service representatives deal with face to face. A custom-designed program can be developed for the organization that provides the peer program with a heads-up for a timely response.

An early intervention analyst can also use the records system to conduct special searches. It may be appropriate to run a check to see how many employees have attended to more than a determined number of sudden-death incidents within a specific period of time. These types of calls on their own may not necessarily be concerning. But, if one individual attends a high number of death calls in a month, it may be time for a peer to reach out to that person.

In police organizations, there is a program, called BlueTeam,[4] that is primarily used by the Internal Affairs or Professional Standards Department for discipline. If the early intervention analyst has access to the program, they may be able to generate information that will be helpful for peer support. (However, any searches using this program must be entirely confidential.) There are several searchable categories that can provide useful information to alert the Peer Support Team that a member may be developing a mental health issue or exhibiting some unhealthy behaviours. These categories are:

- Sick Time - how much sick time a member is taking and if there has been a significant increase or change in the pattern.

- Bereavement or Compassionate Leave - an automatic indicator to reach out to a member.
- Missed Events - such as a scheduled court appearance, paid duty or a special assignment.
- Speed Notifications - Some organizations have vehicles with an automatic notification system that identifies when a vehicle exceeds a certain speed.
- Use of Force Reports - are submitted in police services when a member needs to use a level of force to deal with a threat or to effect an arrest.
- Public Complaints - members of the public filing complaints about the behaviour or attitude of a member.
- Members facing criminal charges or internal discipline.
- Personal Evaluations - significant changes in evaluation ratings.

The idea is to intervene, if there is some reason to believe that a specific behaviour may be related to a mental health issue, and to do so before it is investigated by another department.

DUTY REPORTS

Most organizations have a shift report that is completed by a senior member of the organization at least once daily. In policing, fire and EMS, these are usually done by the duty officer, lead road supervisor, platoon chief or the communications supervisor. It is essential that the peer support coordinator be on the email dissemination list, so that an intervention or confidential contact can be made to anyone involved in a call that raises concerns. These reports are primarily completed for operational reasons; however, they are excellent tools for the Peer Support Team. More often than not, a call of interest to the peer team will be on that report.

PROJECT SAFEGUARD

Many organizations have extra measures in place to protect and safeguard their members. In policing, there is a program known as Project Safeguard that focuses on the wellness of those who conduct investigations that are high risk to cause an operational stress injury. (Among these high-risk areas are: traffic reconstruction, forensic identification, Internet child exploitation, child abuse, homicide, human trafficking and covert operations.)

Similar to those who are peer team members, candidates who work in high-risk areas undergo a written psychological assessment and an interview with a psychologist to determine if the candidate is healthy enough and suitable for the high-risk position. There is an orientation period where the individual can change their mind. There is an annual assessment with the psychologist, as well as an exit interview when they leave the unit. There is also follow-up within a year of the completion of the high-risk assignment.

Programs such as this are the ultimate strategy in terms of being proactive and providing early intervention. Any organization can have a program such as this for their high-risk areas. Organizations are responsible for ensuring their employees do not head into harm's way. The irony is that the very organizations that are developing peer support and CISM teams to deal with the after-effects of work-related injuries are the ones who are sending their members into high-risk and challenging situations.

Psychological Services

Psychological services are an essential element of a wellness and peer support system. The organization is establishing a peer support and CISM system to support the psychological well-being of its workforce. It is crucial to the success of the peer support system that there is clinical direction to ensure peer support is being provided in a safe and appropriate manner.

Each intervention that is undertaken by a peer supporter should be reviewed by a clinician. Trained and experienced peer supporters know what they are doing and are competent to provide appropriate support. They also know when there is urgent need for professional assistance. Many teams will have a weekly briefing to review the interventions that were conducted. During these briefings, the peer lead and the mental health professional will work together to determine if there is anything more that can be done to help the individual. The clinical director may be able to provide advice on a person's behaviour or feelings, and will suggest others ways to assist and direct that individual.

Many large organizations are able to hire a full-time psychologist on staff. Although a competent psychologist can be a significant asset to any organization, they are generally hired as a full-time senior manager. Senior management can be viewed as a pipeline to other managers or the CEO or chief of the organization. This raises many issues about confidentiality and trust which are the pillars of a peer support system.

An alternative is to use a number of mental health professionals under contract to the organization. The psychologist who supports the peer support program can report and take direction from the peer lead. In this way, they are not seen as being part of management. There are a few benefits to having more than one psychologist under contract. The work that the psychologist does for and with the peer support group is different than what a psychologist does as part of the organization's human resources department.

Using a variety of mental health professionals allows an organization flexibility in case one provider takes leave, or becomes ill, or is not providing consistent quality service. Mental health professionals can be used in other areas of the organization for health and wellness files, accommodation strategies and for clinical direction when challenging members with behavioural problems.

Mental health professionals come from various backgrounds and have a history of specialization or expertise in different areas of wellness, for example, addictions, trauma, brain injuries and so on. It is important to remember that a mental health professional, who is consulted and relied on for disciplinary matters, cannot be used in the peer support program. It is essential to maintain the credibility of the peer support program by using objective members on the team.

TRAUMA RECOVERY GROUPS

There is a growing trend to partner peer support with trauma therapy in the form of a trauma recovery group. As an example, Gary Rubie, a retired Peel Regional police officer and the author of *Out on a Cliff*, is the lead peer on the trauma recovery group at Homewood Health Centre in Guelph.[5] As a lived-experience survivor of trauma and addictions, Gary has significant credibility and knowledge. He is instrumental in helping participants, especially first responders, find a path to wellness.

Trauma recovery groups need to maintain confidentiality. Wherever possible, organizations need to support these groups. In fact, organizations with contracted and trusted mental health professionals should be encouraged to initiate groups such as these. Introducing peer support into trauma support groups is helpful because it takes some pressure off the mental health professional. It also provides the mental health professional with some lived-experience perspective when developing strategies to lead the peer to wellness. It can create an amazing partnership.

The strategies and tools presented in this chapter are intended to help the organization in setting up the way in which its CISM/peer support program will work best for its employees.

12

Walking the Talk—The Last Word

The title of this book, *Walk the Talk*, has described the lived experiences of both authors as they travelled on the road to recovery from their work-related traumas. Their stories, which follow in the next two chapters, are intended to send a message of hope to others who have endured the same trauma which resulted in post-traumatic stress. Their stories also describe their experiences in helping organizations create peer support systems.

The authors were both members of police services when they experienced their traumas as a consequence of the jobs they signed on to do. What they were not prepared for was the psychological ramifications of what happened to them after their shooting incidents. Nor were they aware of the fact that their organization did not have any way to support them on the road to recovery. In fact, their organizations had no understanding of what its workforce was up against as a result of these incidents.

This book shows how these two men walked the talk to set up peer support and CISM systems for their mutual police services often against the odds that they might be successful. The authors describe in detail what an organization—or first responder service—needs to know today about ensuring their workplace is both physically and psychologically healthy for its employees or members.

They detail what mental health standards have been developed today and what an organization needs to do to adopt these standards as part of their workplace environment. Then, they walk the organization through what it needs to do to get onside with mental health policies and procedures.

Their journey through their individual lived experiences convinced them that, having walked the talk, they could provide direction and help other organizations, especially first responder agencies and services, to develop programs of peer support. They believe this is the best and most effective way for the organization to provide assistance for their employees to regain mental health.

This boots-on-the-ground book is intended for everyone in the workforce—from top down to bottom up—to create the healthiest workplace possible for an organization's greatest asset—its employees.

13

Brad's Story

Brad McKay and his co-author, Syd Gravel, have over fifty-five years of peer support experience. Both authors have been chosen to lead teams of competent and capable peers with lived experience, along with mental health professionals.

These groups provide advice and suggest training to organizations in need of peer support and trauma management programs. Competent peer support is the conduit that gives first responder organization members the confidence they need to get professional help. They come to these groups seeking help and putting their trust in them. Such a group might well have shortened Brad's road to recovery from his exposure to trauma.

This is his story.

The Trauma Event

As the shift began at the stroke of midnight on 29 September 1984, I was a young twenty-five-year-old constable with just over two years of road experience. I had just paraded at the Richmond Hill Station for my shift. I was assigned to the 235 area, located at the eastern edge of the town of Markham, north of Toronto.

We always paraded standing in a line with our revolvers out of our holsters. We had to show our cylinders, so that the sergeant knew we had bullets in our guns. We also showed our cuffs hooped onto our wooden billy sticks. We wore tunics with a leather cross strap and cross-draw holsters that we called widow-makers because it was easier for the bad guys to get our guns than it was for us to draw them.

It was my turn to buy coffee. Donny and I met on the patrol area border and chatted about buying a home in Aurora—I was saving up—and about our families before going off to our patrol areas. I chatted with the paramedics who were also working the area and we wished each other a safe night.

A call came in that an off-duty police officer needed assistance. Just prior to this call, there had been a report of a man kicking in the front windows of a gym in the same area. The restaurant owner who made the call said that a man was urgently pleading for help.

Because the York Regional Police was a fairly small service in 1984, it was easy to check and discover that no plainclothes officers were deployed in the area, so it was possible that a Toronto officer, or someone else from another jurisdiction, had issued the call. When a call comes in that an officer needs assistance, there is an immediate and rapid response. Everyone goes to assist that officer and everyone headed to the area to find him.

Donny got there first. But, instead of welcoming help from Donny, the man turned on him and fired a shot from what appeared to be a large revolver. Donny fired back but the man escaped and ran toward a busy and crowded tavern. Donny had given good instructions on the location of the man. I pulled up and ran into the bar to find the gunman and another officer—Wayne—on-site.

The bouncers in the bar were shaking. The man had pointed a gun at their heads indicating he wanted to shoot someone. It was dark in places inside the bar with the music blaring and the lights flashing. It was crowded and chaotic.

I spotted the gunman by the bar. He had a revolver out and he was pivoting and pointing it at many people as he stood in a combat position. Those who noticed him were screaming, running and diving under tables, while others were oblivious to the threat. At one point, the bartender threw a credit card machine at his back and knocked him to the ground. He bounced back up to his feet and started making his way toward the raised dance floor.

Wayne and I paralleled him through the bar until he reached and stepped onto the dance floor. There were always people between the gunman and us. He was pointing his gun at us, at patrons in the bar and at the dancers on the stage. Both Wayne and I yelled at him to drop his gun. As soon as the dancers were off the raised dance floor, and as soon as I had a clear and unobstructed view, I shot the gunman. As I learned later, I had severed his aorta.

By this time, several officers had arrived and helped me hold the man to the ground as he was trying to get back up on his feet again. When he had dropped to the ground, so did his gun. The impact broke the handle, revealing a CO_2 cartridge. The gun was not real; it was not a lethal weapon. A CO_2 gun hurts but it cannot seriously injure or kill anyone. Essentially, I had shot an unarmed man.

The man I shot was David, a troubled young man whose stepfather was a Toronto police officer. David looked up to him. Toronto Police had pulled him from the Bloor Street viaduct the year before because he was going to jump and take his own life. He had been in and out of a mental health facility. He had also been charged with setting fire to an apartment.

The Aftermath

ORGANIZATIONAL REACTION AND RESPONSE

Police officers are trained to respond, eliminate a threat, preserve the peace and keep the community safe. It's what we signed up to do. And we are prepared to do what it takes, within the limits of the law, our abilities and our training. What we are not always prepared for is how to face the stress and acute reactions after a traumatic incident.

I was holding it together on the outside, yelling over the radio to rush the paramedics and putting on a brave face as I was expected to do. On the inside, however, I was full of anxiety. It seemed like forever before the same paramedics I had spoken to at the coffee shop arrived in less than ten minutes to treat David who was now unconscious. He was transported to North York General Hospital where he was pronounced dead.

My head was spinning. I was experiencing an enormous amount of guilt, full of doubt and second guessing myself. I was sitting alone on a bench in the bar. My sergeant had seized my gun. The first to check on my psychological well-being was John Lucas, a fellow officer. He sat on the bench with me for about five minutes until the sergeant told him to move away because my statement had not yet been taken. I was driven to the Richmond Hill Police Station where I was left alone waiting to be interviewed formally.

The investigative team was thorough and professional. David's mother had insisted that the detectives deliver a message to me. It was the most significant gift of my entire career. She wanted me to know that she understood that I was doing my job and that she supported me in my actions. This was an unbelievable show of support! I had just shot and killed her son, and she forgave me. Although it was not an easy road, this was a huge boost and helped to accelerate the healing process. Without it, I am certain I would have fallen much harder.

What also helped was that the media took only minimal interest in the event. No media showed up at the scene. They reported on the shooting for a couple of days and during the inquest the following January. Extensive media attention around an officer's actions, especially if it is negative, can amplify the stress reaction after a traumatic event.

PERSONAL REACTION

Police officers are responsible for confronting and eliminating a threat to the safety of others. It can result in a loss of life. It is what police officers are trained to do. Where training has failed is in the mental preparation of officers about what we will experience afterward, that is, the natural reaction a first responder faces after involvement in an unnatural event, in this case, the moral injury of taking a life. (It never occurred to me in the aftermath of the shooting that I may have been used as a tool to commit suicide. I had never heard of the phenomenon of "suicide by cop." It was almost a year later when a colleague shared with me a study on this subject.)

Personally, I felt as if everyone was watching me. No one really knew what to say and, when my coworkers did say something, it was awkward for everyone. One officer slapped me on the back and said, "Good work, killer." When I went to my firearms requalification, the instructor announced in front of the class that I had already re-qualified in the field. Although these were well-meaning attempts by fellow officers at their dark humour, I would have preferred that they not make comments in public but rather speak to me alone.

In 1984, there was no system of psychological support for members of the York Regional Police. There were no psychologists on staff and no employee assistance program. My inspector called me into his office a week after the shooting and asked me if I wanted to go see the Toronto Police Department psychologist. Because I thought he was testing my toughness, I immediately declined the offer.

But I quietly and confidentially sought help and support through my own sources. I was blessed with a strong network of family, friends and a church upbringing. I could never admit at the time that I was suffering or having difficulty because I feared that it would translate into Brad McKay being weak. Instead, I focused all my efforts on trying to show that I was doing all right. I was frightened of the stigma attached to being seen as vulnerable. Often described in my evaluations as quiet and conscientious, I was determined to find my own way and I continued in my chosen career as a police officer.

Developing a Peer Support Network

Nevertheless, I knew I would never make up for the life that had been lost, despite the gift of forgiveness I had been given by one of the parents. I was determined, however, to make a difference in my organization to support members who experienced traumatic events such as the one I had been through.

As a lived-experience survivor, I began lecturing newly hired recruits in their classroom setting. I often found that telling the story repeatedly was almost as traumatic as the event itself. But re-living that event was helpful for the mental preparation of new officers. I also found it therapeutic for me.

In 1989, I cofounded the York Regional Police Trauma Team, the first formal peer support system implemented to assist officers who had been involved in a shooting incident. I never had difficulty finding other officers who had been through a similar experience. After their ordeal, they would be at the York Regional Police Association bar. Consuming significant amounts of alcohol after a traumatic event was seen as a solution for the officer at that time.

My initial strategy then was to show support simply by being present for an officer. I would try to meet with the officer in the days following the event when there was an opportunity there to interact and intervene privately and confidentially to show support. However, I truly believe that peer support and taking care of our own is not something we can do alone. It is a collaborative effort that requires working with others who have the highest level of ethics, standards and skills, and respect the need for utmost confidentiality.

Getting together and supporting each other in a group setting can be very effective. In 1995, I joined with a steering committee to create a multidisciplinary Critical Incident Stress Management (CISM) Team in the York Region. In 1996, when the team was formed, I was assigned co-lead along with the clinical director. Together, with like-minded people and organizations, we now had the ability to make a huge difference in providing support and care to our people. Because we believed in collaboration, the CISM Team served first responders from the police, fire, emergency medical services (EMS) and hospital emergency department staff.

During the early stages in developing this team, I met Dr. Barbara Anschuetz, which was a turning point in my life. She is an energetic, skilled, ethical and effective trauma specialist and, for twenty years, she has been the clinical director for the team. She has invested thousands of hours of her own time in this volunteer position to benefit frontline responders and their families in York Region.

She instilled confidence in me and gave me the tools to develop and enhance peer support programs. She showed me how loyalty, integrity and some hard lessons about boundaries were essential to ensure credibility and trust. She encouraged me to seek further education and training, and sponsored me in becoming a certified trauma services specialist.

In January 2002, we were the co-leaders of a three-element debriefing team that was sent to New York City to assist the New York Police Department in dealing with their trauma exposures after 9/11. We shared the lessons we have learned and have presented at conferences in Miami and Frankfurt, Germany.

The Trauma Centre, a facility located in the hamlet of Sharon, just north of Newmarket in the York Region of Ontario, specializes in trauma recovery and bereavement. The facility serves frontline responders, military personnel and their families. There are over fifteen highly trained and skilled professionals who provide treatment and support under the clinical direction of Dr. Anschuetz.

In its early stages, the centre donated space for the CISM Team. In return, frontline responders from all disciplines formed a work party to help paint and set up the centre. The Trauma Centre is taking great strides to reduce the stigma of mental illness. In fact, it is not unusual to see frontline

Illustration 13.1: Erin's Dad

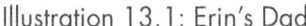

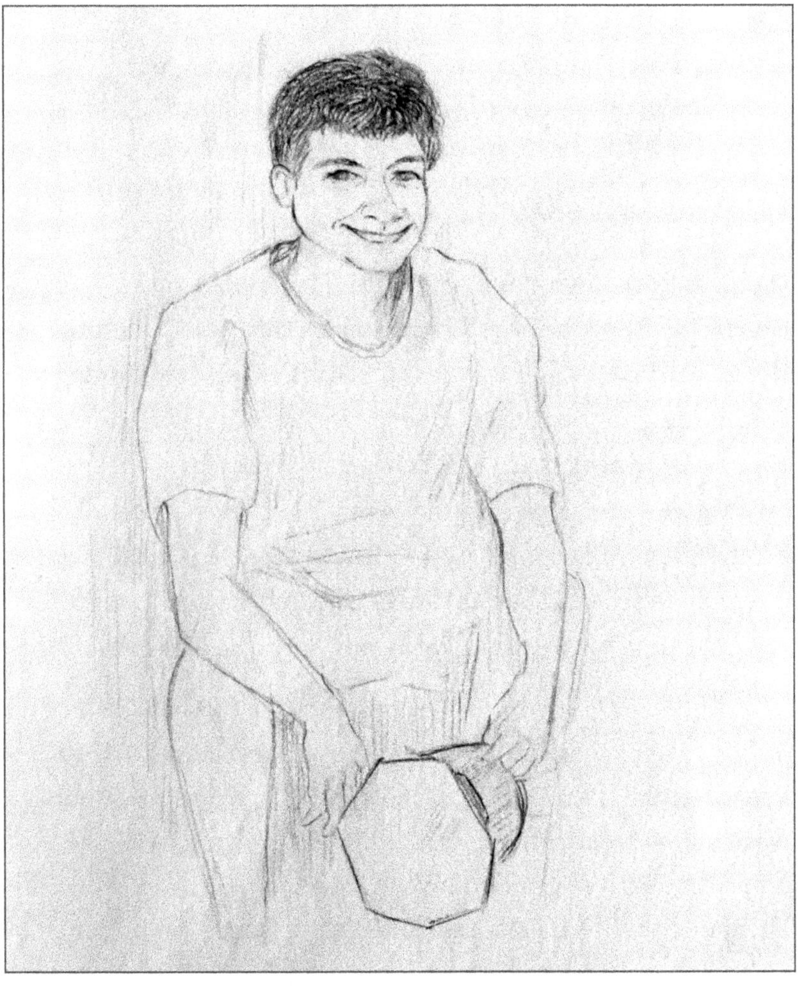

Brad McKay by Erin McKay

responders showing up for their therapy appointments in uniform or to see an emergency service vehicle sitting in the parking lot, safely recharging before going on to the next call.

In 2003, I began a collaboration with The Tema Conter Memorial Trust, an organization created to provide frontline responders with training, education, awareness and support for trauma exposures. After surviving his own journey through trauma exposure, Vince Savoia established a trust to help others like himself to deal with the effects of post-traumatic stress disorder (PTSD).[1] Among many other achievements, he is a pioneer in the peer-driven, peer nomination model of peer support.[2]

Where I Am Today

In 2013, York Regional Police Chief Eric Jolliffe and Deputy Chief Tom Carrique asked me to take a full-time position in the health, safety and wellness area of the service in order to create and enhance peer support systems. This was the first time in my career that I was being paid to perform these duties full-time, which is unique in a police environment. I brought in two others— Beth Milliard[3] and Jen Thompson, a crime analyst,[4] who became an early intervention analyst for the organization. We named the new unit the OSI Prevention and Response Unit.

In 2014, we created an internal peer support team, using the peer nomination model, and welcomed twenty-nine members from many areas of the organization to the unit. We have created other working groups in Ontario and connected with Dr. Jane Storrie and the Psychological Association of Ontario to help psychologists better understand the police personality.

Brad's Story

I met Syd Gravel at a suicide seminar in Niagara Falls, New York, which has led to another turning point in my career. His passion for wellness and compassion for first responders was immediately apparent, so we invited him to be our keynote speaker at the CISM Team family evening.

After thirty-three years of policing, it was time to move on and let others manage the CISM Team.[5] I retired and started a business, 228 Solutions—in honour of the organization and community I served under badge 228. I live in Aurora with my daughters Taylor and Erin, and continue to volunteer with both of the peer support teams I helped to create. I provide professional, clinically supervised peer support at the Trauma Centre. I am also the peer lead at a weekly yoga program for first responders in Newmarket.

I have joined Syd Gravel as co-lead of the Peer and Trauma Support Systems Group at Mood Disorders Society of Canada. It is an honour to be working with him on so many initiatives. Syd is an incredibly passionate man, who has dedicated and donated more time than anyone could imagine to the cause of wellness for frontline responders.

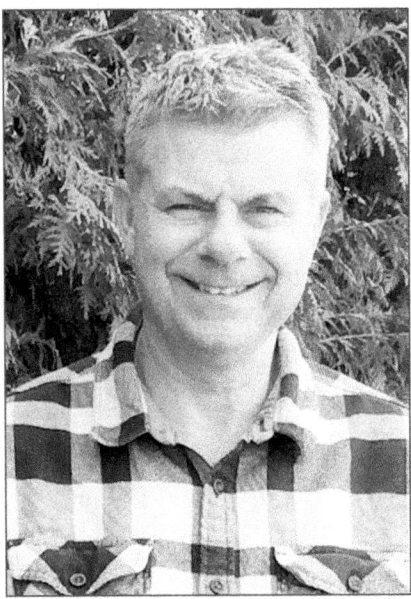

In March 2016, I accepted a senior police advisor position with Badge of Life Canada, a collaborative and valuable resource hub organization that drives police wellness initiatives.

14

Syd's Story

As one of the co-authors of this book, Syd Gravel recognizes that there are many ways to approach peer support management. He is personally well acquainted with the informal peer support structure. To help him lead and develop a team of advisors for a formal trauma management and peer support group, he sought the help of Brad McKay, one of the best in the business. Brad also agreed to co-lead the Peer and Trauma Support Systems Group at Mood Disorders Society of Canada.

Syd fully realizes the impact that peer support—whether formal or informal—has for those who have experienced a trauma-induced injury while doing their job as a first responder. Had there been organizational support and expertise available to him, his decades-long battle with PTSD might have been considerably shortened. Here is Syd's story.

The Lead-Up

Fresh out of college, I worked for a company that was doing survey work along the border of Tanzania and Mozambique. At the time, the Frelimo Revolution was going on in Mozambique. Tanzanians were understandably nervous of any stranger walking around in their forests. At one point, while working in the bush in the middle of the night, I was surrounded and captured by very agitated and aggressive soldiers. My boots were removed and I was told to keep my elbows above my ears. I was marched through the bush at gunpoint—several of them. I was eventually paraded through a village, where the locals lined the road and struck at me with sticks and stones.

When we reached the prison, I was incarcerated and questioned there for ten days. I was suspected of being a mercenary and connected with the Frelimo Revolution. My saving grace was that my captors found only survey equipment in my camp and no weapons, so I was released.

I spent some time in Dar es-Salaam undergoing medical care from the beating I had received while in prison. However, I was young and resilient. I came out of that experience tougher rather than damaged. I spent two more years in Africa surveying in Nigeria, just after the Biafran Civil War, and in various other countries. But I was always nervous and aware of the local political climate and the aggressive way locals dealt with disputes.

Finally, I returned home to Ottawa. But I noticed I had some difficulties in being around large crowds. I also often had restless nights and abused alcohol. Over time, I settled down, cut off my alcohol abuse and started to sleep better. In my mind, this was the end of these experiences and their effects.

After my overseas experiences, I continued to survey in Canada. Most of the upcoming work, however, was overseas in Third World Countries and I didn't want to do this anymore. I applied for and joined the Ottawa Police Service as a constable and was hired in October 1978.

After only one week on the job and while being coached by a senior patrol officer, we were involved in a vehicle pursuit of

Syd's Story

two armed robbery suspects. It was winter. At one point during the pursuit, both of our vehicles went off the road and hit snowbanks. I got out of the patrol car and approached the suspects' vehicle on foot. They had managed to free their vehicle and suddenly I found myself in its path. I dove out of their way and shot at the driver as he drove by me.

By this time, my coach officer had also managed to free the patrol car. We continued our pursuit of the suspects' vehicle. Several blocks later we were able to surround them with the help of other police cars. We managed to arrest both suspects who were unharmed.

I had discharged my .32-calibre Colt weapon at the getaway car. The bullet had gone through the window and then dropped, after bouncing off the suspect's head. No one had been hurt except from flying broken glass. But I was suspended for three days without pay. My superiors considered that my life was not in danger and there had been no need to discharge my firearm. On the advice of the association representative, I pleaded guilty, as the representative said I could have been fired by the police service.

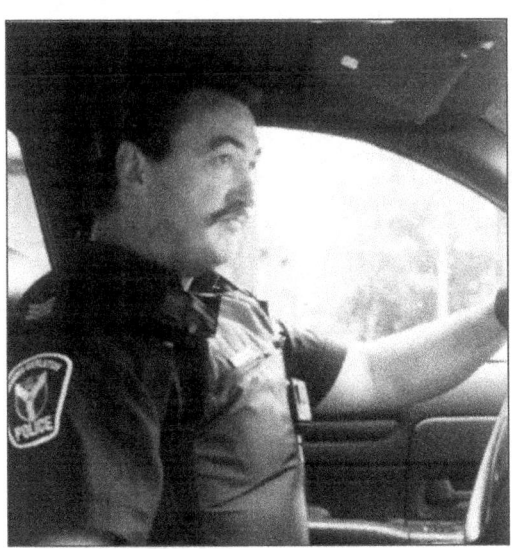

Syd in a patrol vehicle as a member of the Ottawa Police Service.

After the incident and a few days off work, I somehow came through the experience none the worse physically or mentally. It was part of the job. I had experienced one more important lesson, which was that everything I did in policing would be very carefully scrutinized. It was not a bad lesson to learn after only weeks on the job.

Despite these two experiences, I maintained a positive outlook on life. Although I had some difficulties, there was nothing overwhelming or concerning to me about my reactions up to this point in my life.

The Trauma Event

Eight years into the job, while responding to an armed robbery, my partner and I found ourselves in pursuit of a vehicle with two robbery suspects in it. This time I was the coach officer and my partner was a recruit. It did not go well.

We had been advised that a 10-42 had just happened. At that time, any 10-42 call meant that an armed robbery had occurred and we were to assume that the suspect was armed and dangerous. We were expected to prepare and react to the worst possible scenario. Within a few minutes, we were pursuing the suspects, who were in a car.

After the suspects rammed into three parked cars, they were finally forced to stop; the suspect on the passenger side abandoned the vehicle. We pursued him on foot and, during this time, my partner and I gave several very clear and precise commands to the suspects to show their hands where they could be seen. I was worried in that I had not yet established which of the two suspects had a gun, or if they each had a gun, since we had been advised that we were responding to an armed robbery.

Syd's Story

The passenger I was primarily focused on stopped as he stood on the rear end of the car they had crashed into and turned to his left to look at me.

> . . . he had his right hand stuffed into the front of his jeans. I yelled at him several times to show me his hands as we locked eyes. But then he started to turn in the opposite direction toward my partner, who was standing off to the suspect's right side and focused on the other suspect, [who was still in the car.][1]

"As I had . . . not yet determined where the weapon was, I couldn't let him complete that turn."[2] By training, I had made the natural conclusion, in anticipation of the worse possible case, that he was armed with a gun. ". . . I couldn't give the suspect the opportunity to pull out a gun that he may have stuffed down the front of his pants. . . . [I] pointed my gun at the suspect and shot at him to stop him from continuing to turn toward my partner."[3]

> I was prepared to tap off two shots, as I had been trained, but the suspect went down as soon as I fired off the first shot. . . . I heard someone screaming to my right. Then, the suspect I had just shot stood up again and I got ready to fire off another shot. . . . However, it wasn't necessary, as he just stood straight up, then went down again.[4]

The second suspect was still in the car in the driver's seat. He put his hands up where I could see them and gave himself up. I pulled him out of the car and started to place handcuffs on him, when I felt a tap on my shoulder, wost triggered a violent reaction on my part. As I turned quickly, I saw that it was a fellow officer offering to take over the arrest of the suspect. I accepted his help, stood up, backed away and looked around.

I saw my partner running toward the suspect I had shot at and I joined him in the area where the suspect was last seen. At this point, I was not really sure if I had even hit him or if he was simply hiding between the cars. When we got to him, he was laying face down on the ground, rolling from side to side. We carefully turned him over and I saw the wound. I called for an ambulance which had already been dispatched. The suspect still had his hand in the front of his jeans. We unzipped his pants and slowly pulled his hand out. There was no gun.

My breath was knocked out of me. I felt faint and fell back against the car. Oh my, God, I thought, what have I done? The paramedics arrived and I stepped back from the suspect lying on the ground.

THE MIND

Throughout this entire scenario, I felt like I was physically out of sync with time, sound, sight and smell. I remember scanning the area and seeing my partner leaping toward the passenger side of the suspects' vehicle as I ran toward the driver's side. My partner seemed to be moving in slow motion and hanging in the air in between steps. I saw a man standing on the side of the road with a dog on the end of a leash and a lady standing on the front porch of a house, which was located next door to where we were. I knew she was saying something but I couldn't make sense of what it was. Everything was happening in slow motion with moments of real time interspersed. At one moment—and only for a second or so—it all became really strange. I seemed to be watching everything from up in the air ten feet above and behind me like a movie in slow motion. Throughout all this distortion and confusion, I struggled fiercely to think logically and clearly. It became apparent to me that, if ever I truly had to concentrate on what I was doing, it was at this moment; otherwise, I had no control whatsoever.

After shooting the first suspect, all the distortion disappeared. Instantly, everything became clear and precise during the arrest of the second suspect. But once I handed him over to another officer, everything went out of sync again. There were several police cars there, a fire truck and ambulance as well as first responders walking and running around everywhere. There were lights flashing and sirens going off. Yet I had heard and seen nothing up to this point. Now I could hear and see everything for the first time. Just then the logical part of my brain tried to come back to life. I felt physically exhausted, as if I had run five kilometres. I was out of breath, sweating profusely, shaking like a leaf and almost incapable of standing up on my own.

After the paramedics took over helping the suspect I had shot, I leaned back against a patrol car. I was feeling both faint and nauseous, and held myself up only by leaning against the car. I was flashing in and out of the present. Everything being said and done around me was clear and precise one moment. Then for a split second, everything would move in slow motion with sound being slow, low and distorted as well.

I remember the sergeant at the scene approaching me and saying something as he stared at me. But I couldn't make out what he was saying. Then, almost like cotton being pulled out of my ears, I clearly heard him say, "Syd, I will need to take your gun from you." I gave it to him. Then I thought, What happened? I also realized that I was not well, which was an understatement!

The Aftermath

There truly isn't a day that goes by that I don't think about the horror of that moment, a moment when I made the decision to react—to shoot or not to shoot. Then deciding to shoot—having no choice—I learned the shot was fatal. And I found out that the suspect was not armed after all. I always wish that I hadn't been there at all. However, I was and it happened. I can never change that. So, every day, day after day, for more than twenty-nine years now, I continue to doubt there will ever be an end in sight.

Those who investigated the shooting and dissected my decision-making second by second did not find any wrongdoing. My decision to shoot was deemed to be the correct one based on all the facts. Nevertheless, this decision was a marked departure from how I was raised. Nor was it why I joined the police service. I didn't join to cause harm; I was raised wanting to help people, not kill them. I understood the concept of using force if necessary. But I never equated doing this part of the job with the personal and moral conflict it would create in me. The fatal use of force would cause me considerable suffering.

As a result of this incident, the injury to my brain was indeed a physical one. Based on everything we know about trauma today, this is not in doubt. The chemicals that flow freely within the brain to help it stay healthy and smooth running were thrown out of balance. This imbalance happened instantly from the moment that I went from using a logical clear-thinking brain to one that had switched to the primitive reactions of fight or flight.

I could tell things were different in the seconds—that felt like minutes—during the incident itself. Sound was distorted. For example, in the split second as I pulled the trigger, it sounded like popping corn. A split second later the same sound now came to me as if I had shot off a canon. My visual perception changed as well, as I watched smoke and flames slowly come out of the end of the gun barrel. I saw a huge tree in the way of my line of sight. I was worried about how I could use the tree to both protect me but, at the same time, get around it to pursue the suspect. In truth, the tree was only half an inch in diameter. As I interacted with the suspect, it seemed as if time stood still.

Once these parts of my brain, which controlled my instinct to survive, went into overdrive, they didn't turn off easily. I found myself locked into a world of fear, anxiety, panic attacks, irritability, nightmares and paranoia. These were only a few of things I found myself struggling with for weeks after the incident. My brain was locked in the fight or flight position and interfering with the other parts of my brain that would allow me to think calmly, clearly and logically; to feel safe once again; and to return to live as I had before.

Little did I know then that this would never happen. Psychologically, my personal and well-established emotions, thoughts and behaviours had been thrown out of balance, compared with my usual emotions, thoughts and behaviours. I was a mess and there truly didn't seem to be a way out of it as I tried to fix it all on my own.

The Downward Spiral

After the incident, I tried to reason my way out of it. I spent hours and hours pacing the living room floor, night after night, after everyone else in my family had long gone to sleep. I was trying to logically work my way past the barrier that blocked my ability to understand what had happened out there. I was trying to feel safe and secure again in my own environment. I kept going over the event, asking myself hundreds of times, Did I miss something? Did I react too quickly? There was never an answer for me. The point was that no matter how justified the act to shoot was deemed to be, I felt broken inside. I couldn't figure out how to fix myself so I could stop thinking about what had happened.

My staff sergeant at the time suggested that I go home and have a few drinks; things would be okay the next morning. His was the Korean War experience, so I took his advice to heart. Over the next few weeks, I tried drinking myself into a stupor several times. I thought this would not only close down my body but also shut my brain off. But I still woke up. Only now I found myself drunkenly pacing the floor with even less control of my thoughts than when I was sober. Things were worse than ever.

I tried to self-medicate by popping pain and anti-inflammatory pills hoping that my body would be forced to sleep. But my brain wouldn't shut down and I always woke up anyway. Now I would pace the floor lethargically. This didn't work either.

I tried using both medication and alcohol together and this just scared my wife. She ended up staying awake all those nights, watching over me as I laid in bed kicking and lashing out, and shouting out all night long. Just being in bed with me was not safe for her. This wasn't working.

Throughout this time, I continued to work as a patrol officer. For some reason, once I put on the uniform, I was able to lean on my training, the workplace environment of strict regulations and the professional expectations of me in uniform to do what I was trained to do. Somehow I was able to convey to everyone at work that everything was fine.

Finally, after several weeks—leading into months—of living like this, I reached a dark and exhausting place where suicide seemed the best and only option left to me. I had held on as long as I could. Now it was time for the pain to end.

My wife, however, had determined that this was not going to happen. She knew that somewhere within the mess of a man that she now lived with, there was the man she had once loved, and married and had children with. She needed to find him in me again and I needed to find him too. But all my attempts had failed so far.

Personal Reaction and Spousal Support

I wasn't ready to admit that I needed help, although I realized I was really screwing things up on my own. My wife, on the other hand, knew that I would not be able to recover on my own. Unknown to me, she reached out for help. First she called the police station and pretty much was given little help. Then she called the police association and was transferred immediately to the president, who listened carefully and told her that he didn't know what he had to offer. However, he said he would find out and call her back. Within half an hour, he did and gave her the name of a psychologist, experienced in dealing with Vietnam veterans.

Once she had connected with the psychologist, she found out he was willing to see me right away. She tearfully and, with a broken heart, made it very clear to me that I had no options. I needed help and she had arranged for me to get it. I had no choice but to accept the psychologist's help.

From the moment I met with the psychologist, he explained to me that my reactions were completely normal reactions to an abnormal situation. He advised me that there were things I could do for myself, with his help and direction, that would lead me out of this spiral of self-destruction. I felt a great sense of relief. I vividly remember the weight of fear and anxiety lifting from my shoulders and I actually did feel lighthearted. At the same time, I also began to visit our family doctor to include him in what was going on in my life; he was ready to help in any way he could.

Now the journey to recovery began. It took time and not every step forward stayed a step forward. Every now and again I would fall back—but never as far back as I had been before. With every step forward, I became stronger. And with each and every one of those steps that I took, my wife walked along beside me. In fact, she carried me through most of the journey. I could not have done this on my own and I know this now. My wife was so proud of me. We consciously and intentionally took this journey together. We had to fall in love all over again, since I was now someone new, someone who was not the person she knew before the shooting.

At some point, which I don't remember, I realized I actually had a full night's sleep. I couldn't believe it. Although the damaging event never left my mind, I was learning to live with it rather than struggling to deny it. I realized that I would have to live with the horror of that moment forever. But I could put some techniques and thought processes in place now that would allow me to move on despite the memory. I knew I could conquer this. I had just needed help getting there.

There were some setbacks, however. As the years went on, something was still wrong and I couldn't figure out what it was. Despite the support I was receiving, I still struggled with the decision I had made that fatal day. One time in particular,

I was deeply depressed and struggling with suicidal thoughts. After Judy had left for work and the children had gone to the babysitter, I went to the basement and planned my death. But Judy had realized that there was something off with me; she called a family friend to come and talk to me. He arrived at the precise moment when I planned to end my life. I broke down and admitted my thoughts. Once again, I was placed under medical care.

The Moral Injury

The most significant issues I had to address were anger and the lack of trust I had in my workplace. It's hard to trust an organization when you are being investigated by other members of the workforce as a criminal for having done what they asked of you. In communications with me, a correspondent shared the following: " In some cases, the failure of 'The System' is worse than the injury caused by the original incident. When the people who are supposed to help you, turn you away, doubt your story, or drop the ball, the result can be devastating."[5] He goes on to point out, "And the deeper that sense of injustice, the more persistent the physical and psychological injuries will be, the greater the anger and bitterness . . . and the more ridiculous words like 'acceptance' and 'forgiveness' will sound. 'Letting go' won't seem like much of an option."[6]

In 2015, Dr. Jonathan Douglas, a psychologist, pointed out to me that this phenomenon of anger and mistrust that I had gone through is now being referred to as sanctuary trauma.[7] Sanctuary trauma is one of the major reasons why members of first responder services—and war veterans—who are already suffering from a work-related trauma, continue to struggle to regain their mental health.

It took me six years to get past my anger and distrust of the work environment. But, when I finally did, it was such a relief. What helped was reading and thinking deeply through philosophical stories such as this one by Tanzan (18??-1892) who "was a Buddhist monk and professor of philosophy at the Japanese Imperial University (now the University of Tokyo) during the Meiji Period. Considered a Zen master, . . . [the] following is one of his most famous stories called *The Muddy Road*:

> Tanzan and Ekido were once traveling together down a muddy road. A heavy rain was falling. As they came around the bend, they met a lovely girl in a silk kimono and sash unable to cross at an intersection.
>
> "Come on, girl," said Tanzan at once. Lifting her in his arms, he carried her over the mud.
>
> Ekido did not speak until that night when they reached a lodging temple. Then he could no longer restrain himself. "We monks don't go near females," he told Tanzan, "especially not young and lovely ones. It is dangerous. Why did you do that?"
>
> "I left the girl there," said Tanzan. "Are you still carrying her?"[8]

"Letting go of a problem is always difficult."[9] However, I slowly came to realize that no matter how angry I was, I could not stop the beauty of a sun rising or the stars from shining. "Eventually, I came to realize that the guy who was hurting me the most was me. I stayed angry far too long. Once I realized that I was harder on myself than anyone else was, I was more capable of facing the challenges of trying to get along with others and letting go.[10] Once I addressed the anger, healing progressed quickly.

Finally, in 2016, it all started to make sense to me. I discovered through the work of Dr. Jonathan Shay, a clinical psychiatrist who has spent over twenty years working with the U.S. Department of Veterans Affairs, that there is such a thing as moral injury. From various readings and browsing websites, I have found one definition for this injury: "Moral injury is the damage done to one's conscious or moral compass when that person perpetrates, witnesses, or fails to prevent, acts that transgress their own moral and ethical values and codes of conduct."[11]

Along with learning about this injury, I also came to the realization that there are three pillars to good mental health. The first is the physical injury which requires medication. The second is the psychological injury that requires therapy and the third and, often forgotten pillar, is the moral injury, which deals with the soul, the core being and our personal spirit.

It is this moral injury that sometimes feeds our anger the most. Everyone around you is treating you like a hero for having the courage to do what you had to do. Outwardly, you show appreciation for their supportive comments but, inwardly, you feel emotionally broken. Managing this deep-rooted anger and this contradiction in emotions is truly difficult to do by yourself. This is why having a group of peer supporters to lean on, individuals who have walked in similar situations, is absolutely crucial.

Peer Support

Dr. Shay believes explicitly in the value of peer support. He states:

> Peers are the key to recovery—I can't emphasize that enough. Credentialed mental health professionals like me have no place

> in center stage. It's the veterans themselves, healing each other, that belong at center stage.
>
> We are stagehands—get the lights on, sweep out the gum wrappers, count the chairs, make sure it's a safe and warm enough place for the peers. . . .[12]

Peer support is the foundation through which lived experience connects with empathy for those who have been traumatized. Peer support gets the medical or psychological help needed for an individual who reaches out. Peers support an individual through the healing process and offer reassurance and guidance. Once an individual is strong enough, peer supporters let the individual go without any obligation for the support that was offered. No single mental health service on its own can provide everything that is needed. All services and support need to work as one for the benefit of the sufferer.

The informal peer support group that was started among Ottawa police officers involved in shootings in 1988 still exists today. It has been instrumental in helping hundreds of officers over its many years of existence. If it hadn't been for this peer group, it would have been considerably more difficult for my family and me to recover.

Over time, with the help of family, friends, doctors and peers, I started the journey toward positive growth. Even with the informal peer group that I had joined, there were times when we struggled in spite of all the help that we offered each other. I still would suffer from debilitating bouts of depression or experience a paralyzing anxiety attack. But I was learning to manage these situations with medication, therapy and peer support.

Where I Am Today

At the time of the shooting, I was a constable. Over time, the police service recognized my ability to handle myself and, after eighteen years on the job, I was promoted to sergeant on patrol. Then I was promoted to staff sergeant in charge of recruiting and training for the service. I was invited by the United Nations to take part in a short peacekeeping mission with the Pearson Peacekeeper's in Nigeria. Subsequently, I was nominated by my peers and the Canadian Association of Chiefs of Police and inducted as a Member of the Order of Merit (M.O.M.) for Police. I retired after thirty-one years as a proud member of the Ottawa Police Service.

On my retirement, I wrote and published my story in the book titled, *56 Seconds*. I followed this up with another entitled, *How to Survive PTSD and Build Peer Support*. Some people say that it helps to write your story. I'm not so sure I agree with this. I tell my story to those who are curious and make it sound like reading a book. But what many don't realize is that, in the telling, we are reliving all the pain, the emotions, the anxiety, fear, horror and loss of control. It all comes back to haunt us again. Even writing this chapter is throwing me into an emotional roller-coaster ride again. Nevertheless, I receive many requests for

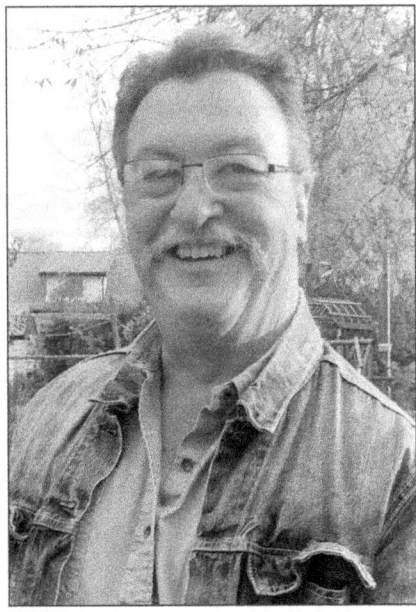

assistance to develop informal peer support groups as a result of my writings and I am forever grateful for that.

I also talk about trauma survival, resilience, trauma management and moral injury. I especially enjoy speaking to families of first responders and trauma survivors. I talk to students who are interested in pursuing careers as first responders or working in the fields of health and wellness. My wife travels with me when I speak to make sure I stay grounded as I speak from the heart and, sometimes, it can set me back a few steps. But I have learned to address those dark moments, when they flash into my life, by using techniques that work for me. I now control the demon that lives within me and my work as a peer is only just beginning.

In 2012, I was contacted by Peter Platt to help him develop a resource webpage to support municipal and provincial police officers, and their families and civilian employees. I was pleased to help him establish the Badge of Life Canada. In 2016, Badge of Life Canada, under the stewardship of Bill and Lynne Rusk, held three one-day workshops on post-traumatic stress. They plan to continue this work and I will continue to support them.

In March 2014, I developed a training curriculum, based on the Mental Health Commission of Canada guidelines for selecting and training peers. Later that year, I joined the Mood Disorders Society of Canada (MDSC) as an advisor for peer support. MDSC also asked me to work with them in the management and training of peers for a police service in Ontario.

Under the lead of Captain Vicki Ryan, I also volunteer to run peer support workshops monthly for Soldiers Helping Soldiers, a peer-driven group that reaches out to homeless veterans.

On a personal note, I love my wife, Judy, very much. We have been married for over forty years. We are happily and busily retired with three wonderful grandchildren who love us dearly.

To all those who suffer from work-related trauma, life is worth living and we will be there to help.

Notes

PREFACE

1. 680 News, "Following Toronto Officer's Death, Attention Turns to Better PTSD Assessment," Posted on 5 February 2016; 1:22 p.m. at www.680news.com.
2. John M. Violanti, PhD, *Police Suicide: Epidemic in Blue*, 2d ed. (Springfield, IL: Charles C. Thomas, Publisher Ltd., 2007).

CHAPTER 1 PROTECTING SOCIETY'S PROTECTORS THROUGH PEER SUPPORT

1. André Marin, Ombudsman of Ontario, *In the Line of Duty* (Toronto: Office of the Ombudsman of Ontario, 2012), p. 136.
2. Ibid., p. 87 as cited from Note 20 on p. 31 of the report.
3. Ibid.
4. Mental Health Commission of Canada.
See mentalhealthcommission.ca/topics/stigma
5. Mood Disorders Society of Canada.
See https://mdsc.ca/stigma/elephant-in-the-room-campaign/
6. Canadian Mental Health Association. *See* www.cmha.bc.ca

CHAPTER 2 ASSESSING AN ORGANIZATION'S AWARENESS ABOUT WORKPLACE WELLNESS

1. *Guarding Minds @ Work (GM@W)*. ©2012 Centre for Applied Research in Mental Health and Addiction (CARMHA). All rights reserved. (http://www.guardingmindsatwork.ca/info) This resource was commissioned by the Great-West Life Centre for Mental Health in the Workplace and funded by Great-West Life Assurance Company.
2. From "The 13 Psychosocial Factors in GM@W" by J. Samra, M.

Notes

Gilbert, M. Shain & D. Bilsker, Centre for Applied Research in Mental Health and Addiction (CARMHA). All rights reserved.
3. Ibid.
4. Canadian Standards Association (CSA), *National Standard of Canada for Psychological Health and Safety in the Workplace* (Ottawa: CSA, 2013.)
From: http://www.mentalhealthcommission.ca/English/issues/workplace/national-standard
5. — and the Mental Health Commission of Canada (MHCC), *Assembling the Pieces: An Implementation Guide to the National Standard for Psychological Health and Safety in the Workplace* (Ottawa: CSA and MHCC, 2014).
6. Mood Disorders Society of Canada (MDSC), *Workplace Mental Health: How Employers Can Create Mentally Healthy Workplaces and Support Employees in Their Recovery from Mental Illness* (Guelph: MDSC, 2014).

CHAPTER 3   GETTING MANAGEMENT ONSIDE

1. Sylvio (Syd) A. Gravel, *Workplace Diversity—How to Get It Right* (Ottawa: Budd Publishing/Syd A. Gravel, 2014), p. 102.
2. Ibid., p. 103.
3. Ibid., p. 104.
4. Ibid., p. 75.
5. Ibid., p. 76.
6. Ibid., pp. 68-72

CHAPTER 4   ORGANIZATIONAL PRE-HIRING PREPAREDNESS

1. Sylvio (Syd) A. Gravel, M.O.M., *How to Survive PTSD and Build Peer Support*, Rev. Ed. to *56 Seconds* (Ottawa: Budd Publishing/Syd A. Gravel, 2013), pp. 7-10.
2. Institut de recherche Robert-Sauvé en santé et en sécurité du travail, "Predictors of Posttraumatic Stress Disorders in Police Officers: Prospective Study R-786. *See* www.irsst.qc.ca

Notes

CHAPTER 5   ORGANIZATIONAL SUPPORT FOR FAMILIES

1. The study can be viewed on a Ted talk video.
2. *See* www.businessinsider.com/robert-waldinger-says-3-things-are-the-secret-to-happiness, 29 December 2015.

CHAPTER 6   MIDDLE MANAGEMENT LEADERSHIP

1. This level of management among first responder services includes sergeants, staff sergeants and duty inspectors in police services; captains and platoon chiefs in fire services; shift supervisors in paramedic organizations; nurse supervisors and doctors in emergency departments.
2. Both authors are retired staff sergeants and understand the role that middle managers can take in leading the organization.
3. Behavioural changes may include: increase in the amount of sick leave, chronically late when normally early or punctual, appearance is sloppy rather than neat, angry when normally calm and composed, etc.
4. Department of National Defence, "Road to Mental Readiness." *See* https://www.forces.gc.ca/en/caf-community-heatlh-services-r2mr/index.page
5. Ibid.
6. *See* https://www.mentalhealthcommission.ca/English/catalyst-jan-2015-r2mr
7. Ibid.
8. The International Association of Chiefs of Police, *Suicide Prevention: A Guide for Supervisory Staff* (Alexandra, VA: IACP). *See* www.theiacp.org)
9. *See* https://www.livingworks.net/programs/safetalk/

CHAPTER 7   DEVELOPING A CRITICAL INCIDENT STRESS MANAGEMENT (CISM) TEAM

1. George S. Everly, Jr., PhD, C.T.S., and Jeffery T. Mitchell, PhD, C.T.S., "A Primer on Critical Incident Stress Management" from https://www.icisf.org

Notes

2. T. Snelgrove, "Debriefing under Fire," *Trauma Lines* 3 (2, 1998), 3, 11 and B.E. Bledsoe and D. Barnes, "Beyond the Debriefing Debate: What Should We Be Doing?" *Emergency Medical Services Magazine* 32 (Dec 2003): 60-68.

3. *See* https://www.trynova.org

CHAPTER 8   DEVELOPING PEER SUPPORT TEAMS

1. *Merriam-Webster's Collegiate Dictionary*, 10th ed., s.v., "empathy."

2. Sanctuary trauma is also known as betrayal trauma. This type of trauma occurs when an individual, who thought he or she was safe and supported within the organization in a time of need, discovers that the organization—and their colleagues—are not trustworthy or supporting them at all. They become angry and bitter, and find it difficult to trust anyone, especially those in a position of authority in the organization.

3. Sylvio (Syd) A. Gravel, MOM, *56 Seconds* (Ottawa: Budd Publishing/Syd A. Gravel, 2011), p. 43.

4. ___. *How to Survive PTSD and Build Peer Support* (Ottawa: Budd Publishing/Syd A. Gravel, 2013), p. 121.

5. Gravel, *56 Seconds*, p. 43.

6. Ibid., pp. 43-44.

7. Ibid., p. 45.

8. Ibid., p. 48.

9. This is due to the generosity and support of York Regional Police Chief, Eric Jolliffe.

10. For more information, *see* André Marin, Ombudsman of Ontario, *In the Line of Duty* (Toronto: Office of the Ombudsman of Ontario, 2012).

11. Lived experiences may include: surviving a serious illness; dealing with an addiction or the suicide of a family member or close friend; coping with difficult children or a family member diagnosed with a mental or life-threatening illness; surviving the death of a spouse or a child or some mental health challenge such as depression or anxiety; experiencing workplace conflict or discipline; caring for elderly ill parents; or dealing with the homicide of a family member or a colleague.

Notes

CHAPTER 9   STAFFING CISM AND PEER SUPPORT TEAMS

1. One thing both authors learned as they journeyed through the world of peer support was that, as constables, they were viewed and trusted as equals by the front lines of their respective organizations. However, as they were promoted up the ranks, they noticed that the higher the rank, the less credibility they retained with the front lines. The good news for the authors is that they are still asked to provide peer support and more so since they have retired.

2. The MMPI 2 revised edition from Pearson is utilized by many recruiters in policing organizations. The Trauma Symptom Inventory -2 by PAR is used to evaluate acute and chronic posttraumatic symptomatology.

3. Mental Health Commission of Canada, *Guidelines for the Practice and Training of Peer Support* (Ottawa: Mental Health Commission of Canada, 2012), p. 22.

4. One of the authors, Brad McKay, has been on interview panels with the Toronto Paramedic Service and the Vaughn Fire and Rescue Service.

5. Bruce was also a deputy chief with York Regional Police.

6. Beyond the Blue was developed by the Calgary Police Service. The program has been adopted by York Regional Police.
See yorkbeyondtheblue.com; calgarybeyondtheblue.com; and canadabeyondtheblue.com

CHAPTER 10 ORGANIZATIONAL TRAINING FOR CISM AND PEER SUPPORT TEAMS

1. Mental Health Commission of Canada, *Guidelines for the Practice and Training of Peer Support* (Ottawa: MHCC, 2013).
See www.mooddisorderscanada.ca

2. ©2014-2016 LivingWorks Education.
See https://www.livingworks.net/asist

3. Ibid. *See* https://www.livingworks.net/programs/asist

4. International Critical Incident Stress Foundation, Inc. (ICISF) or Canadian Critical Incident Stress Foundation.
See https://www.icisf.org/individual-crisis-intervention-and-peer-support/ or www.ccisf.info (*See* Mission Statement.)

Notes

5. ___. *See* https://www.icisf.org/individual-crisis-intervention-and-peer-support
6. ___.*See* https://www.icisf.org/group-crisis-intervention
7. The Tema Conter Memorial Trust. Source: http://www.tema.ca/#!maners/c1wle. Used with permission.
8. International Critical Incident Stress Foundation (ICISF). Used with permission. *See* https://www.icisf.org/advanced-group-crisis-intervention/
9. ___. *See* https://www.icifs.org/suicide-prevention-intervention-and-postvention/. Used with permission.
10. National Organization for Victim Assistance (NOVA). *See* http://www.trynova.org. Used with permission.
11. Association of Traumatic Stress Specialists (ATSS). Copyright 2016. All rights reserved. *See* https://www.atss.info/index.php/certification. Used with permission.
12. Ibid.

CHAPTER 11 HOW A CISM AND PEER SUPPORT SYSTEM CAN WORK

1. Both authors have had considerable success in collaborating with different organizations.
2. Mood Disorders Society of Canada, *Workplace Mental Health: How Employers Can Create Mentally Healthy Workplaces and Support Employees in Their Recovery from Mental Illness* (Guelph: Mood Disorders Society of Canada, 2014), p. 29. *See* www.mooddisorderscanada.ca
3. The International Critical Incident Stress Foundation (ICISF) has compiled a list of the top ten incidents that first responders are exposed to, which may cause acute stress or an operational stress injury. These are: a line-of-duty death, a serious line-of-duty injury, suicide by a fellow emergency worker, a disaster or major multi-casualty incident, significant events involving children, incidents involving relatives or known victims, prolonged incidents (especially those with a life loss), excessive media interest, emergency service activity that results in the death of a civilian and any high-power

event. For more information, *See* https://www.icisf.org

4. Blue Team is a digital platform used to document critical incidents for police services. This is one of several product lines available from IAPro, a professional software standards company.
See https://iapro.com

5. Gary Rubie, *Out On A Cliff*. Published 11/01/2014. *See* www.outonacliff.com

CHAPTER 13   BRAD'S STORY

1. Vince Savoia was a paramedic in 1988 when he attended at the scene of the brutal murder of Tema Lisa Conter in Toronto. He battled the symptoms of PTSD as a result of the traumatic event.
2. Both Vince Savoia and Brad McKay have interviewed peer prospects for the Toronto EMS and for Vaughan Fire and Rescue.
3. Beth had completed her master degree, writing a paper that dealt with the benefits of psychologically safeguarding members in high-risk units.
4. Jen has significant analytical skills and extensive knowledge, education and experience in dealing with mental health challenges.
5. The team is led by Todd Snooks, along with Mechtild Uhe, the clinical director.

CHAPTER 14   SYD'S STORY

1. Sylvio (Syd) A. Gravel, MOM, *56 Seconds* (Ottawa: Budd Publishing/Syd A. Gravel, 2012), p.4.
2. Ibid.
3. Ibid.
4. Ibid, pp. 4-5.
5. Personal communication in 2009.
6. Ibid.
7. Dr. Douglas became president of the Ontario Psychological Association in 2016.
8. Gravel, *56 Seconds*, pp. 39-40.
9. Ibid., p. 40.
10. Ibid.

Notes

11. Syracuse University, The Moral Injury Project. *See* http://moralinjuryproject.syr.edu/about-moral-injury/ *See also* http://www.goodtherapy.org/blog/psychpedia/moral-injury
12. Jeff Severns Guntzel, Guest Contributor, "Beyond PTSD to 'Moral Injury'." *See* http://www.onbeing.org/blog/beyond-ptsd-to-moral-injury/5069

About the Authors

STAFF SERGEANT (RET'D) BRAD MCKAY, C.T.S.S.

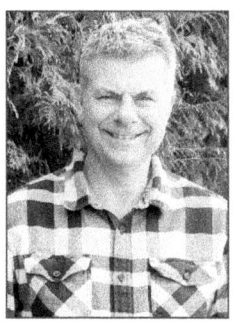

Brad McKay retired in 2015 after thirty-three years of service with the York Regional Police (YRP). In 1984, he was involved in a shooting incident that resulted in the loss of a life. At that time, there were no formal peer support or mental health programs available at YRP, so he processed the event on his own with help from his network of family and friends.

In 1989, he co-created a trauma team to support YRP members involved in police shootings. He transitioned this team into the York Region Critical Incident Stress Management Team in 1996. He is an advisor to the executive and an alumni team lead. The York CISM Team is unique and ground-breaking as a multidisciplinary team in that it supports all first responder services including police, fire, paramedic and emergency department staff. To enhance wellness at YRP, he started the Operational Stress Injury Prevention and Response Unit in 2013; he also created the York Regional Police Peer Support Team in 2014.

As a Certified Trauma Services Specialist with the Association of Traumatic Stress Specialists, Brad has responded to and coordinated hundreds of interventions for frontline responders and their families. Brad has been asked to appear on TV news to provide the first responder perspective.

Currently, Brad is providing clinically supervised peer support for mental health professionals in York Region and is the peer lead for a weekly yoga group for first responders. Brad is proud and honoured to join Syd Gravel in co-leading the Peer and Trauma Support Systems (P.A.T.S.S.) Team. This is a team of highly skilled, trained, experienced and professional peer and mental health experts from across Canada. Many of these professionals have volunteered countless hours to support frontline responders.

Brad recently joined Badge of Life Canada as a senior police advisor and volunteers on two peer teams. A family man, Brad is a community-minded energetic advocate for wellness and peer support.

STAFF SERGEANT (RET'D) SYLVIO (SYD) A. GRAVEL, M.O.M.

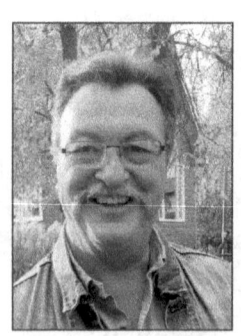

Syd Gravel is a former staff sergeant with thirty-one years of experience with the Ottawa Police Service. He is one of the founding fathers of Robin's Blue Circle, a post-shooting trauma team of peers, established in 1988.

Syd is a more than twenty-eight-year PTSD survivor and has been a peer supporter since 1988. In 2007, he was nominated by his peers and the Canadian Association of Chiefs of Police and inducted by the governor general for the Order of Merit in Policing in Canada.

Since his retirement, he has devoted all his time and energy to speaking on developing resilience and resistance to trauma and setting up peer support systems. He has written and published *56 Seconds* and *How to Survive PTSD and Build Peer Support*.

In 2014, Syd developed a trail-blazing curriculum for the certification of peers in Canada, based on the guidelines and practice for the selection and training of peers developed by the Mental Health Commission of Canada.

Syd is currently co-leading the Peer and Trauma Support Systems (P.A.T.S.S.) Team for the Mood Disorders Society of Canada. He is a lead facilitator for peer workshops for Soldiers Helping Soldiers in Ottawa. The peer work focus is on helping homeless veterans.

He has developed the content for the three days of peer training for the Transitions to Communities Project for the Mood Disorder's Society of Canada. He has also developed the content for an on-line trauma management course for Simon Fraser University in Vancouver.

Syd is a board director for Badge of Life Canada. In 2016, he was nominated by the Mental Health Commission of Canada as a Canadian Champion of Mental Health.

What Others Are Saying

ABOUT BRAD MCKAY

Neil Orr, Ret'd Constable, Former Secretary, York Regional Police Association and York Regional Police

> *Finally, the masses will see and read what many have known for years. Brad is the total package when it comes to sharing lived experience trauma and putting it into terms that everyone will understand. Brad's character and reputation have been synonymous with excellence throughout his policing career. Always there with an offer of a coffee, a shoulder to lean on or an ear to listen, Brad is the consummate "go to guy." By sharing his knowledge and experience, Brad will inspire and validate those who have struggled with, or those who love someone who has struggled with, PTSD. Brad was my "go to guy" and I am proud to call him my friend. After reading this book, I'm sure you will see how lucky I am!*

Thomas Carrique, M.O.M., SBStJ, MA, Deputy Chief of Police, York Regional Police - Operations Branch

> *Throughout his thirty-three-year career with York Regional Police, Staff Sergeant Brad McKay was highly respected as an exceptional police officer who excelled on the front line and as a detective. A police leader, who truly led by example as a mentor, team-builder and action-orientated advocate, Brad was committed to the development and well-being of others. His encouraging leadership style and relentless dedication to the service of others were instrumental in establishing the York Region Critical Incident Stress Management Team and our Peer Support Unit. Brad's career has left a legacy that will ensure the best possible care and support are available to the members of York Regional Police and other emergency services personnel who have dedicated their lives to the safety and security of our citizens.*

What Others Are Saying

Dr. Beverley Bouffard, Registered Clinical Psychologist, Toronto/Aurora, Ontario

What instantly struck me about Brad, when I first met him at an interview at the York Regional Police several years ago, was his warm smile and genuineness, and his firm and unwavering passion for mental health awareness, prevention and intervention in policing. Well, it didn't take long to realize that my radar was right on!

Working with Brad over several years, it was easy to see why he had earned such deep respect from his colleagues, from his platoon mates and the executive command—for thirty-three years! A not-so-easy task in police organizations! Why? With Brad, what you see is truly what you get. His passion for early intervention, critical incident debriefing and peer support came from his own lived experiences. No one can better "walk the talk."

Building a peer support team/network in an old-school organization is no easy feat. Brad did it from the ground up creating the York Region Critical Incident Stress Management Team in 1996, when mental health issues were but a mere whisper in a hallway, suppressed and buried for fear of professional recrimination. Since that time, Brad has literally responded to and coordinated hundreds of interventions for frontline responders and their families. In the often static world of policing, he's truly a pioneer and innovator!

His sheer wealth of experience with interventions for officers and their families, and building resilience and suicide prevention, is unparalleled. As a consultant to the Mood Disorders Society of Canada and an ongoing consultant to the executive command at the YRP, he is truly the real deal!

In fact, people who have worked with him over many years will describe him just as I saw him that first day as "sincere, compassionate, solid, competent, sharp, respected, kind-hearted." But he's also steady as a rock and will be there for you in a heartbeat. He's incredibly quick-witted, so watch out. He can banter with the boys/and girls but is always respectful of his position.

Finally, as a mentor and educator, Brad really walks the talk on resilience. He really aces the concept of work/life balance. When he glows about his daughters and shows you his latest motorcycle trip photos—with his father—you'll see what I mean!

What Others Are Saying

ABOUT SYLVIO (SYD) A. GRAVEL

Dan Bowers, Ret'd Sergeant, Ontario Provincial Police

Sylvio (Syd) is a sought-after speaker and has delivered presentations to diverse organizations on a wide range of topics, including breaking down barriers in addressing mental health in the workplace, suicide prevention, building resilience to trauma, and helping families of those afflicted with PTSD.

He helped develop a web-based continuing medical education course for primary care physicians and specialists, directed at diagnosis, clinical approach to treatment and stigma reduction for those suffering from PTSD.

Having known Syd for a number of years, I would say that what most distinguishes Syd's character is his unfaltering availability and willingness to help his colleagues and their families at any time of the day or night. His tireless, voluntary efforts put toward awareness, education, support and effective treatment of PTSD in first responders are exemplary.

Ed Mantler, Vice-President, Programs and Priorities, Mental Health Commission of Canada, Ottawa

Since his retirement, Syd has devoted all his time and energy to promoting and protecting mental health, building resilience in the face of trauma and promoting peer support systems within first responder organizations.

By sharing his personal experience as a PTSD survivor, Syd provides hope to other officers who have suffered psychological injuries from traumatic events faced during their policing career. Syd provides a unique contact-based training experience. He is an excellent resource for policing organizations looking to implement new strategies and a tireless leader, continuously driven to improve the quality of life of first responders living with, or in recovery, from a mental illness.

Sylvio (Syd) exemplifies the values, dedication and passion that all individuals involved in mental health or other fields should aspire to by being both selfless and relentless in the pursuit of improved quality of life for first responders living with a mental illness.

What Others Are Saying

Dr. Manuela Joannou, BSc. (Hon), M.D., CCFP (EM) is a Family Physician and Emergency Medicine Physician

> *Syd is an exceptional man. He has been tirelessly expending great effort in championing awareness of PTSD in the police world, as well as educating the public, setting standards for peer support systems and, most importantly, being available at all hours of the day and night to support individuals in need.*
>
> *Syd was inaugurated into the world of PTSD by lived experience twenty-eight years ago. He writes of his own journey of personal struggle and healing in his book* 56 Seconds *which has been well acclaimed. He is also the author of the book* How to Survive PTSD and Build Peer Support *which in my view should be the textbook for any policing or first responder organization charged with the responsibility of establishing an effective peer support system.*
>
> *Syd researches the field of PTSD in Canada relentlessly and keeps many interested parties up to date on developments and news items. He has educated me and many others thoroughly on the scope of the problem, what organizations are doing, what works and, most importantly, how addressing the moral injury aspect of PTSD is the most important component of promoting effective healing.*
>
> *He has delivered countless lectures, provided course material and participated in too many projects and reports for me to mention.*
>
> *It is my fervent belief that it will be pioneers like Syd, who are so willing to give generously of themselves, that will be the ones to catalyze the necessary quantum shift required to bring about real change to the mental health services delivery in our society. Syd truly is a champion of mental health, peer support and suicide prevention in Canada.*

www.ingramcontent.com/pod-product-compliance
Lightning Source LLC
Chambersburg PA
CBHW050244170426
43202CB00015B/2904